DØ777776

opportunities to care:
the pfizer guide to
careers in nursing

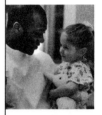

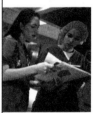

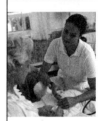

A MUST-HAVE GUIDE THAT
PROFILES THE LIFE AND WORK
OF NURSES IN THE FIELD

Book Editor:
Reeva Friedman
Director of Operations
Global Outcomes Research, Pfizer Inc.

The Pfizer Career Guide Series Editor:
Salvatore J. Giorgianni, PharmD
Director/Team Leader, External Relations
Pfizer Pharmaceuticals Group, Pfizer Inc.

Opportunities to Care: The Pfizer Guide to Careers in Nursing
Assistant Editor: Marlene Lipson

Other Pfizer Career Guide Publications:
Full Preparation:
The Pfizer Guide to Careers in Pharmacy

Embracing Your Practice:
The Pfizer Guide to Careers for Physicians

Advancing Healthy Populations:
The Pfizer Guide to Careers in Public Health

ISBN 0-9602652-0-1

Printed in the United States of America

table of contents

table of contents

acknowledgements

Special appreciation goes to all of the many nurses in the field who were willing to put time aside to talk about their daily experiences on the job and the time and skill required to get them where they are today. Through their everyday work and accomplishment, these people are just some of the many crusaders currently paving the way for all those entering the profession.

Melissa Allan, RN, BSN

Donna Brassil, MA, RN, CURN

Kathryn Changas, RN

Colleen Conway-Welch,
   PhD, CNM, FAAN

Bonnie Daly, RN

Karen Desjardins, RN, GNP

Judy DiFilippo, RN

Nancy English, PhD, APN, CS

Harriet R. Feldman,
   PhD, RN, FAAN

Judy Flynn, RN

Mary Foley, RN, MS

Maureen Furnari, RN

Donna Gaffney, DNSc

Linda Gibbs, RN, MBA

Catherine Gilliss, DNSc, RN, FAAN

Katie Green, RN, BSN

Susan M. Huff, RN, BSN

Virginia Klunder, RNC, MA

Marilyn Kaufmann, PhD, RN

Elaine Larson, PhD, FAAN, CIC

Timothy Lehey, CRNA

Lisa Kane Low, PhD, RN, CNM

Elizabeth A. McFarlane,
   RN, DNSc, FAAN

Kathy Magdic,
   RN, MSN, ACNP-CS

Ellen Mahoney,
   RN, DNSc, CS, CARN

Marie Ann Marino, EdD, RN, PNP

Ron Martin, RN

SueAnn Montfort, RN, CHPN

Barbara Neilson, RNC

Jane Newman, RN, MPH

Mary Olszewski, RN

Major Matthew M. Ruest, RN, MS

Debra A. Sansoucie,
   RN, EdD, CNNP

Patricia Seifert,
   RN, MSN, CRNFA, FAAN

Sue Sherman, RN, MS

Kimberly Thomas, RN

Jan Towers,
 PhD, CRNP, NP-C, FAANP

Bill Thompson, RN, BSN, CCRN

Diane Vogelei, RN, MSN, ANP-C

Deborah S. Walker,
 DNSc, CNM, CS, FNP

Agatha Wilkos, RN

Finally, and most importantly, the expertise, guidance and everyday support from Mary O'Neil Mundinger, RN, Dr PH, Dean, and Centennial Professor of Health Policy, Columbia University School of Nursing was instrumental in the development of this book. Thank you.

a letter from pfizer

Reeva
Friedman
Director of
Operations,
Global
Outcomes
Research

Dear Nursing Student:
Congratulations. You have chosen a career that is both noble and gratifying, one in which you will play a unique and valuable role in patients' lives.

As you join the ranks of the country's more than two million registered nurses — the nation's largest health care occupation — you will face an array of exciting career choices. Your work can focus on the heart, the mind, or any part of the body. As a nurse you can choose to work in a busy emergency room, clinic, surgicenter, laboratory, or nursing home — anywhere in the world. Nurses advocate for their patients and teach them. Nursing care extends beyond their patients to their patients' families and communities. There are more choices now than ever before.

To help you evaluate these possibilities, Pfizer has joined with other health care leaders to create this guide to nursing careers. In the pages that follow, nurses in various practice areas share their experiences — how they got started, the hurdles they encounter every day on the job, and their hopes for the future. It is important to point out that the 31 practice areas detailed in this book are simply a glimpse into the universe of nursing specialties and subspecialties. There are many, many more equally exciting pathways from which to choose.

As a leading, global health care company, Pfizer is pleased to provide this tool for nurses to help them prepare for an essential and exciting role in patient care around the world. We commend you for your choice and wish you much success and happiness in this great adventure.

Sincerely,

Reeva Friedman

Reeva Friedman

the future of nursing

By Mary O'Neil
Mundinger, RN,
Dr PH,
Dean, and
Centennial
Professor of
Health Policy
Columbia
University
School of
Nursing

This book is designed to introduce you to the opportunities in the rich field of nursing. We hope this book will help you evaluate the different specialties available to you by sharing the stories of those in the field. Whether your interests steer you to a primary care nurse practitioner career, to pediatric palliative care, to the fast-paced atmosphere of an urban trauma center, or to looking after the health needs of children in an elementary school, you will be joining a profession at the peak of its power. Never before have nurses had such potential for a full scope of practice and direct decision making.

We, who have been nurses for decades, celebrate the choices you will have in today's nursing environment. We're also pleased to have been the pioneers

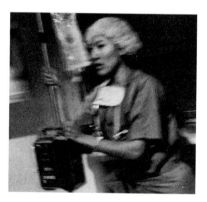

for many of these new professional roles. And we know you, too, will continue to sustain and advance nursing's unique and valuable contributions and be pioneers for the generations of nurses yet to come.

Since Florence Nightingale wrote nursing's name in the history books over a 150 years ago, the world has changed dramatically, and nursing right along with it. It seems like only yesterday when nurses stood shoulder to shoulder with physicians as both professions learned the value of such a simple thing as washing their hands before treating each patient. They stood together and watched as the new drug "penicillin" effectively fought what up until then had been deadly infections.

But today, nurses face new challenges — and we meet them with our modern day arsenal. For example, by 2020, more than 20 percent of our nation will be "seniors." Thanks to contemporary medical care, those over 85 are already the fastest growing age group in the country. This, however, has left us holding a double-edged sword. Yes, people are living longer, but because they are, we are experiencing an increasing number of chronic

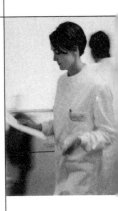

and acute health problems. This stresses a healthcare system already hard pressed to provide efficient and effective continuing care to the current population.

And the graying of America isn't all that's occurring. We are also becoming a nation more diversified than any other in the world. The consequence is a medical community challenged with accommodating a myriad of ethnic groups, each with different values, attitudes and traditions, in a way that provides equal care to each person. Translators are routinely summoned to emergency rooms when a non-English-speaking patient arrives in acute distress; some hospitals have started to specialize in, and indeed advertise, "non-transfusion" surgery to accommodate certain religious beliefs; families are increasingly encouraged to stay in the room overnight with an ill child or a spouse.

Moreover, the rapidity with which the planet is shrinking has created another double-edged sword. International travel means individuals can sometimes bring back infections and disease to a community that has not experienced them before. We all know that new epidemics can blanket an area quickly, creating a need for us to be well prepared to fight them. On the other hand, cures for these non-indigenous diseases may well come from the growing medical collaboration between different cultures and healthcare systems outside the United States.

Computer technology — spawning new forms of clinical diagnosis and treatment — has advanced as an answer to these growing problems. Advanced technology will only grow more prominent in medicine as gene mapping further advances the understanding of disease and the development of new methods to treat and prevent them. Thanks to digital technology, diagnostic consultations and monitoring, treatment of the sick can now, if necessary, be provided miles away from the individual being cared for, further shrinking the planet while offering high quality care for all.

Already, nurses are at the forefront of a rapidly changing healthcare environment with new and unforeseen challenges constantly emerging. Cutting edge technology and ever-changing patient care settings are now taken for granted in most of the developed countries of the world. As diverse populations of individuals live longer with their diseases or disabilities, new specialties are arising to meet these needs. Many of the new nursing opportunities available to you are in sub-specialties, some of which — pain management, for example — were unheard of even a year ago.

What does all this mean? Consider where we have been and where we are headed; consider the unfolding opportunities to be part of the world of science and the world of people. Today's nurse is more than ever the conduit of care — the person who keeps the human (and often humane) focus of medicine on the patient. Today's nursing landscape offers many opportunities, challenges and rewards. With this framework, we hope that you too will embark on a career with which to embrace the opportunities, grow from the challenges, and most importantly, share in the many fulfilling rewards, just as your predecessors have.

Mary O'Neil Mundinger, RN, Dr PH is the Centennial Professor in Health Policy and Dean of the Columbia University School of Nursing. She is an elected member of the Institute of Medicine of the National Academy of Sciences, the American Academy of Nursing, the New York Academy of Medicine, and a 1984–85 Robert Wood Johnson Health Policy Fellow. Dr. Mundinger currently sits on the board of directors of United HealthCare and Cell Therapeutics, Inc.

Dr. Mundinger is the founder of Columbia Advanced Practice Nurse Associates (CAPNA), the first nursing school faculty practice where nurse practitioners hold commercial managed care contracts and are compensated at the same rate as primary care physicians.

Dr. Mundinger holds a BS cum laude *from the University of Michigan and a doctorate in public health from Columbia University School of Public Health. In 1996 she was awarded a Doctor of Humane Letters (Honorary) from Hamilton College. In 1995 she was the first nurse to be honored and profiled by the University of Michigan as a distinguished alumna.*

career planning and your resume

One of the unique things about nursing is that there is no one career path. Once you receive your RN license, many career pathways are open and there's virtually no limit to the number of roads you can travel.

The U.S. Department of Labor says the average employee will change jobs seven times in a lifetime. Nurses do not necessarily move more often, but they probably move more easily. Nurses passing the national RN exam receive a state RN license, which can be easily endorsed by other states as needed. Nurses can also move among many different specialty areas by learning new content and skills at various points in their careers. This is accomplished by taking refresher courses, continuing education courses, employer training and orientation and academic course work.

By Colleen Conway-Welch, PhD, CNM, FAAN, FACNM, Nancy and Hilliard Travis Professor of Nursing, Dean, Vanderbilt University School of Nursing

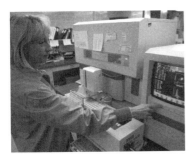

My career is a good example of the flexibility that is inherent in nursing. I graduated with a Bachelor of Science in Nursing degree (BSN) in 1965 from Georgetown University and then spent four months in Syracuse, New York, as an operating room scrub nurse. From there it was on to Hawaii for a year of nursing in a labor and delivery unit and then to San Francisco to run an emergency room. Next, I went back to graduate school in Washington, DC, and supported myself by doing private duty nursing for patients recuperating from surgery.

My travels continued for a number of years. For example, as part of my graduate school program at Catholic University of America in Washington, DC, I became a certified nurse midwife in a training program at the Catholic Maternity Institute in Santa Fe, New Mexico. After that, I moved to Los Angeles to be a clinical nurse specialist in maternity nursing; then on to New York City to the National League for Nursing to write exams that measure nurse achievement and performance. From there, I moved to the State University of New York Downstate Medical Center in Brooklyn to work as a maternity faculty member; then to Georgetown University School of Nursing in Washington, DC, as a parent-child nursing faculty member and associate dean for curriculum. With stops along the way in California (I taught in the graduate program in women's health at California State

University, Long Beach) and Colorado (I ran the graduate program in nurse-midwifery at the University of Colorado), I finally landed in Tennessee. I have been the Dean of Nursing at Vanderbilt University for 17 years and every day new and interesting opportunities come my way.

My story may be a bit unique but not at all atypical. An RN license is a license to practice nursing for the rest of your life. It's an invitation to retrain or retool and to pursue hundreds of pathways in the profession. You can teach or be an administrator, join insurance companies or do research, stay at the bedside or be a trauma helicopter nurse. You can create and control your own destiny.

First and foremost, education frees you. It gives you a lot of flexibility, and a master's degree and PhD give you even more. Additional schooling is a useful investment that not only keeps you current but also gives you many options. Only about seven percent of nurses in this country have a master's

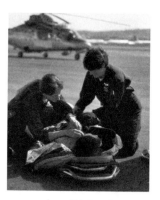 degree and fewer than one percent have a doctorate. As you can imagine, there's enormous opportunity at the upper levels of nursing. As my dad used to say, "Shoot for the top — there's more room."

I obtained my doctorate relatively early — at 26. I'd urge you to get it early, to make the sacrifices when you're young and energetic. Even if you're not so young, I still urge you to advance your education in any way you can. I would also encourage you to make the process efficient. I never took a doctoral course that didn't relate to research I had to do for my dissertation; I maximized everything I did to count twice (if not three times); that allowed me to proceed rapidly up the educational ranks.

My dad was in road construction, so we moved around a lot. I attended seventeen schools by the time I was in the seventh grade. That experience taught me to take risks because I had no choice. I had to figure out quickly how I would be perceived by new people. What I learned worked well for me in building my nursing career: Be flexible and put forth the extra effort. Do the extra work that calls you to the attention of the people in positions

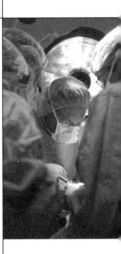

who can open doors for you. The kiss of death for career advancement is being the faculty member, student or employee who will not extend herself or himself without extra consideration or compensation.

Other career-enhancing advice: Get early experience in specialties that require intensive "24/7" time commitments, such as labor and delivery or the emergency room. You need to learn early how to arrange your personal and professional life while being on call, experiencing staffing shortages or managing schedule changes.

Nursing opens up the world to you; take advantage of it! Experience nursing in small, rural, hospitals and big city hospitals, in clinics and in other multiple practice settings. No one school or situation is able to impart every piece of knowledge you'll ever need. Be comfortable and seek out lifelong learning experiences.

The final bit of advice: When job hunting, include references from the chief nurse and chief medial officer in your organization. Use words like "interdependent," "team" and "interdisciplinary" instead of "autonomous." The latter term is a turn-off to some physicians and other healthcare professionals. If you switched jobs fairly often, use terms that indicate that you wanted to gain as much experience as possible in as short a period of time as possible. In your resume, don't do anything eccentric. Your potential employers will judge you by the quality of what you've done, not by the quality of the printing. Also, since many agencies scan resumes by computer for key words, include words like "senior," "interdisciplinary," "skilled," and "experienced" in your cover letter and resume.

Colleen Conway-Welch is a Professor and Dean at the Vanderbilt University School of Nursing and a fellow at the American Academy of Nursing and American College of Nurse Midwives. She holds honorary doctorates from the University of Colorado (1999); Georgetown University (1997); and Cumberland University (1996). She received the NYU School of Nursing Distinguished Alumni Award in 1999. Conway-Welch has been awarded the Nancy and Hilliard Travis Endowed Chair in Nursing at Vanderbilt in 2000 and is a member of the National League for Nursing Accrediting Commission for 2000–2003. She served on the National Bipartisan Commission on the Future of Medicare in 1998–99, and the Advisory Council of the Agency for Health Care Research and Quality (now Agency for Research and Quality [AHRQ]) from 1997–2001.

By Virginia
Klunder,
RNC, MA,
Senior Manager,
Quality
Assurance,
Worldwide
Safety,
Pfizer, Inc.

Few careers in this life offer the rewards, stimulation and diverse opportunities of nursing. But sometimes we stumble over the pebbles in our path
and momentarily lose sight of these benefits. After two decades of nursing,
I've seen plenty and I would like to offer a bit of advice — knowing full
well that most of it you will learn for yourself at some point along the way.

1. **Never stop learning.**
   Education doesn't stop with the degree you've last earned. To be a
   valued member of the nursing community you must continue your
   education, both formal and informal. Don't stop with an associate's
   degree or BS. Go on to get an advanced practice degree, even if it
   means going part time one night a week to do it. Healthcare can be
   very complex, with information coming at us so fast that we must
   absorb it and be ready to meet the challenge.

2. **Maintain a "can-do" attitude.**
   Once you "step up to the plate," opportunities and rewards will come
   to you. Volunteer to do the next admission, work an extra shift or float
   to another unit that needs you more. When asked, say yes if you can.
   It not only demonstrates that you're a team player, but will help you
   learn new skills and make you more marketable. It will be reflected in
   performance reviews for sure, and you may even be tapped by management for special projects.

3. **Listen, and I mean really listen, to your patients.**
   Early in my career as a pediatric nurse, parents would often tell me in
   very unspecific terms that something was wrong with their child. My
   first impulse was to reassure them and get on with things. I remember
   one time I stopped and explored the concerns of a mother who told me
   her infant was fainting. My first thought was that babies don't faint.
   Probing further, it turned out that the infant was having seizures.
   Mothers often know best and so do patients themselves. As a new
   nurse on a medical-surgical unit I brought a batch of pills to an elderly
   woman who singled one out. "I should get a white pill, not a yellow
   one," she repeated adamantly. Because she was so insistent, I went back
   to her chart and sure enough, the physician had lowered her dosage
   that morning. I realized I should never second-guess a patient — they
   have a vested interest in themselves.

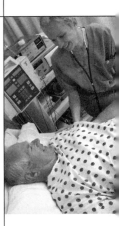

4. **When you don't know something admit it.**
In my career I've seen nurses invent answers to questions they did not have answers to and manipulate medical equipment to try to make it work — sometimes at a disadvantage to the patient.

5. **Recognize that stoical patients still feel pain but manage it differently.**
Members of certain cultural communities who don't verbalize their pain and discomfort are often overlooked. Learn to understand how different cultures handle pain. You may unintentionally under-medicate certain patients because of their no-pain attitude. For instance, infants cry and fuss in response to pain, so nurses often try to pacify them instead of administering medication. Sometimes this works and sometimes it doesn't. And older patients, often labeled as "moaners and groaners," can be shortchanged when they are classified as such.

6. **Don't just treat the patient — treat the family.**
If a partner or other family members are present, include them in the care, assuming, of course, that the patient wants that. This is extremely important with resuscitation and end-of-life situations. During resuscitation efforts, instead of escorting family members out of the room, encourage family to stay, if circumstances permit it, and watch to see that everything possible is done and the patient's wishes are kept in mind.

7. **Vent, vent, vent.**
Nurses are very much affected by positive and negative outcomes and need opportunities to release stress. Utilize debriefing sessions that allow everyone to ventilate feelings and frustrations, especially after failed resuscitation efforts. I've always cried with families but been able to let go — to relinquish my job as a nurse when I go home. That has worked for me, especially in the pediatric ICU where I have lost a good many patients. Remember to develop coping mechanisms and to care for yourself first and not let the lives of patients overtake your own life.

8. **Respect is earned, not automatic.**
   If you want it, you have to consistently project a professional manner. Dressing and looking the part is part of it. Nails must be trim and clean, hair short or tied back. Cleanliness, confidence and a smile help patients know you are professional — and that you respect them and expect respect from them.

9. **Manage the expectations of your patients, which means anticipate and plan for the unexpected.**
   Make sure they know who you are and what you're there to do for them. Everyone wears scrubs nowadays and sick patients can't tell or remember who is who. If you've told Mrs. Jones not to eat because she's having surgery — and a food tray comes and she eats because she doesn't remember the instructions — this does not mean Mrs. Jones was non-compliant. It means the situation was not managed well. Get patients to be your partners. Include them in your plan of care.

10. **Remember why you became a nurse — even on very difficult days.**
    Think about your reasons. Mine are an innate need and desire to help society and make the world a better place to live in. I live nursing every day.

Virginia Klunder practiced bedside nursing for 22 years before moving into the pharmaceutical industry. Her current title is Senior Manager, Quality Assurance, Worldwide Safety, Pfizer, Inc.

planning your career path

I have been in nursing since 1967, and along the way my career has taken twists and turns that I could not have predicted at the start. I have seized opportunities and learned from them. I have not always been clear on what was ahead. How can you know which steps to take as you are getting started? Here are some tips that come from my experiences.

By Catherine Lynch Gilliss, DNSc, RN, FAAN, Dean and Professor, Yale University School of Nursing

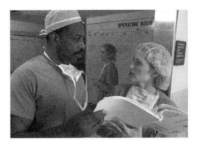

I was not sure I wanted to be a nurse. I did know I wanted to go to college and I began as a nursing major with a music minor. When I entered Duke University for a basic degree in nursing, I wondered whether I actually wanted to be a social worker. It was not until late in my junior year, when I became very involved in clinical work, that I realized that nursing was for me and that psychiatric nursing was where I wanted to be. By then I had given up my music courses, which required more time than I could find. My many interests were becoming focused on one area: clinical nursing.

How did I know this was the right choice? A careful look at my abilities and values helped me sort this out. I am very social and it was important for me to be working with people. I like solving problems, and as I became more engaged with nursing I saw that the practice of nursing involved the use of ideas to solve practical problems. Now that I have been involved in graduate and professional education for over 25 years, I understand that professional education is all about preparing society's problem solvers. I also wanted to contribute to society through service. Nursing met each of these needs. The moral of this experience: If you find an area that matches your values and taps your skills, you can develop a fulfilling career.

My first job after college helped me to determine what I would do next. As is sometimes true in life, the lessons from that experience were largely negative. I worked in a hospital where most of my co-workers had worked for many years. They were angry and bitter people who felt no power to improve their situation or that of the patients for whom we cared. My own youthful idealism was met with scorn and sometimes sabotage. I learned it was important to find a healthier environment, where people were positive, ideas and practical results mattered and where I could continue to learn and grow. After one year I returned to graduate school.

I owe much to those who have mentored me. In my basic degree program, one faculty member counseled me and supervised me in some extra experiences. In graduate school, my faculty advisor was generous with her time and insights. In my doctoral program and while working as a faculty member, still others have shared their caring and wisdom. Being mentored is a treasure, but requires that you be open to sharing your concerns and needs. Although no one person is able to help with all the needs you will have, I have found many people along the way. Be open to being helped.

In 1978 I was awarded a coveted fellowship by a private foundation, but it meant that I would have to relocate to another city. I would live away from

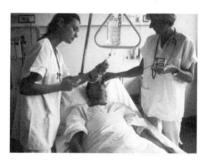 my husband and nine-month-old daughter for nearly a full year; coming home every 10 days for about four days and then heading back again. My husband and I decided that we could manage this and deal with the invasive public queries about our living arrangement. (Some well-meaning people even asked how I could abandon my daughter, as if her father were not capable of caring for her on a daily basis.) I took the fellowship; my career interests and possibilities grew geometrically and my daughter was always happy to see me on my trips home. Sometimes, you just have to do what's important to you. In the end, the decision to accept the fellowship was mine. That year allowed me to transition from psychiatric nursing to primary care. The support I received at home made the whole year possible and rewarding.

Despite the fullness of my career, much of my life's satisfaction and many of my most important life lessons have come from my family. As a wife and the mother of two, I have experienced the frustrations of too little time and competing priorities. Know what is important to you and make the time for it.

Finally, don't be intimidated by other people's life paths. It's easy to assume when you look at the life work of others that they always aspired to be where they are today. Many of us got started without knowing exactly where we were going. I never planned to be a dean or a writer. What I did was take advantage of opportunities that presented themselves to me. Be open to the opportunities as they happen; don't think you need a plan for everything or can anticipate every eventuality. This will also help you to be content and focused on what you are doing. For one of life's great lessons is to know you are satisfied when you are.

Catherine Lynch Gilliss is Dean and Professor at the Yale School of Nursing in New Haven, Connecticut. She has been a Professor and Chair of the Department of Family Health Care Nursing at the University of California, San Francisco and worked at several other universities since 1974. She is a Fellow in the American Academy of Nursing and on that group's Board of Directors. She has been selected for competitive fellowships in primary care by the Robert Wood Johnson Foundation and the United States Public Health Service. An author of over 100 papers, she has received the American Journal of Nursing Book of the Year Award and the Pediatric Nursing Book of the Year Award for one of her co-authored books. She served as a Regent at the University of Portland and in 1995 was named Outstanding Nurse Practitioner Educator by the National Organization of Nurse Practitioner Faculties.

By Mary Foley,
RN, MS,
President,
American
Nurses
Association

the role of the nurse as
part of the healthcare team

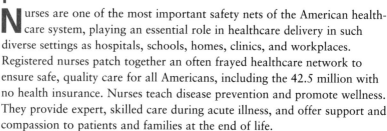

Nurses are one of the most important safety nets of the American healthcare system, playing an essential role in healthcare delivery in such diverse settings as hospitals, schools, homes, clinics, and workplaces. Registered nurses patch together an often frayed healthcare network to ensure safe, quality care for all Americans, including the 42.5 million with no health insurance. Nurses teach disease prevention and promote wellness. They provide expert, skilled care during acute illness, and offer support and compassion to patients and families at the end of life.

The nursing profession has evolved significantly in the past 100 years. The old hierarchical structure of healthcare has given way to a collaborative environment that enhances patient care and increases job satisfaction. Today's nurse is an indispensable partner to all healthcare professionals. The nursing profession weaves the science of nursing with the art of compassionate care.

A good nurse requires critical-thinking skills, in-depth knowledge of pathophysiology and other sciences, and the ability to develop and implement nursing interventions that improve a patient's health and life. The compassion of nursing comes every day, with every touch of a nurse's hand and every extra moment that the nurse listens. It can make a world of difference in a patient's ability to recover. Nurses can be a main source of support. When patients face life-altering diagnoses, it is truly a privileged position.

In some areas, nurses are at the forefront in healthcare delivery. Advanced practice registered nurses (APRNs) play a key role in rural areas and inner cities, which often lack vital healthcare services. Indeed, pediatric nurse practitioners and nurse-midwives emerged as accepted specialties because of the shortage of physicians willing to work in rural and economically depressed areas. APRNs are running primary health clinics across the country and their success can be evidenced by the federal government's continued funding of the Community Nursing Organizations (CNOs). CNOs are nurse-operated programs serving Medicare beneficiaries in home- and community-based settings under contracts that provide a fixed monthly capitation payment for each beneficiary who elects to enroll. CNOs increase benefits, help manage costs, and improve the quality of life for patients, clearly demonstrating what a primary care-oriented nursing practice can accomplish.

No matter what environment they work in, registered nurses are first and foremost patient advocates. In fact, many enter the profession because it affords them the opportunity to work closely with patients. Nurses regard

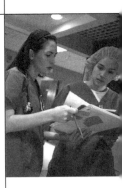

patients and their families as integral members of the care team and believe it is vitally important for patients to be informed and involved in their care so that they understand their treatments. Because they generally spend more time with patients than do other members of the healthcare team, nurses are ideally positioned to advocate for their patients' needs and rights.

The opportunities for nurses are as bountiful as they are diverse. Never before have nurses been able to match their interests, skills, and abilities so closely with a specialized area of practice. There are opportunities for nurses who enjoy writing, who are interested in technology, or who want to lead the charge in the political arena. In many areas of the country, new graduates can begin their careers in emergency and critical care units, as well as in the operating room. Opportunities are boundless for nurses looking to combine traditional care with complementary therapies, such as therapeutic massage and biofeedback.

The nursing profession does include its share of challenges. Cost-cutting in the past decade has resulted in inadequate and inappropriate nurse staffing at a time when patient acuity has increased. In addition to cutting nurse staffing, many financial planners have sought to cut costs by replacing registered nurses with unlicensed personnel. There's historical precedent for this: Unlicensed assistive personnel (UAP) were developed to assist RNs during World War II. While we, as nurses, support their presence as aides to nurses, we do not view them as qualified substitutes for nurses. We also fervently believe that every patient deserves care from a licensed nurse. A major concern is the rapid aging of the nursing workforce, which is expected to lead to a critical shortage of nurses after 2010.

We need to view these challenges as opportunities to reconstruct a healthcare system with cost-efficient plans for excellent care. In the past year, the American Nurses Association (ANA), its state nurses associations, and individual nurses across the country have made progress in addressing workplace concerns. Through workplace advocacy and, in some cases, collective bargaining, nurses have secured workplace protections and an enhanced decision-making role in healthcare. These in turn benefit patient care.

Professional organizations such as the ANA are committed to examining the best practices across the country to help determine nurses' roles in the healthcare system of tomorrow. For example, the Magnet Hospital

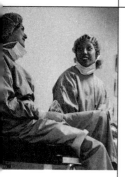

and Long-Term Care programs, developed by the American Nurses Credentialing Center, recognize facilities that have put a premium on nursing care. In these facilities, nurses' expertise and skills are recognized as being integral to the delivery of healthcare.

Never before has there been a time of such opportunity in professional nursing. On every unit and in every setting across the country, nurses are making a difference in the lives of patients, the profession of nursing, and the healthcare industry. If you are looking for a career that will enable you to truly touch the lives of others, you need look no further — nursing can be your opportunity to make a difference.

Mary Foley is on leave from Saint Francis Memorial Hospital in San Francisco, where most recently she was Director of Nursing and Chief Nurse Executive. Previously she served as a medical-surgical staff nurse at Saint Francis for 17 years, was on the faculty of San Francisco State University School of Nursing and was the Assistant Director of Ambulatory Care Review at the New York County Health Services Review Organization. A registered nurse for more than 20 years, Foley has been active in the health-care policy arena, and has served on the California Tuberculosis Elimination Task Force in the Department of Health Services, the Mayor's HIV Task Force for San Francisco and California's RN Special Advisory Committee on the Nursing Shortage for the Department of Consumer Affairs. She also consulted on the Training for the Development of Innovative Control Technology (TDICT) project to prevent exposure to blood through better design and evaluation of medical devices and equipment.

Foley received her nursing diploma in 1973 from New England Deaconness Hospital School of Nursing, her Bachelor of Science in Nursing in 1976 from Boston University School of Nursing in Massachusetts, and her Master's of Science in Nursing Administration and Occupational Health from the University of California San Francisco.

ethics, regulations and standards

By Jan Towers,
PhD, NP-C,
CRNP,
Director of
Health Policy,
American
Academy
of Nurse
Practitioners

The nursing profession is guided by a resolute set of self-imposed and professional standards of practice that began with Florence Nightingale. Over the years, these standards have extended across the profession as nursing practice has grown into the highly skilled and indispensable profession that it is today.

The profession is legally regulated by the State Board of Nursing in each state and professionally guided through standards of practice established by its members. Regulation by State Boards of Nursing guarantee that nurses have passed the national nursing board examination (NCLEX) and have adhered to the educational requirements set forth. Nurses cannot legally practice in the United States without a license issued by the State Board of Nursing in the state in which they desire to practice.

Nursing Boards are comprised of nurses from multiple disciplines, consumers, and selected government officials representing the health interests of the state. The members are generally appointed by the governor and are charged with developing and implementing regulations regarding the practice of nursing in their state. Nurses who violate the Nurse Practice Act by practicing outside the scope of their license or who do harm to patients can lose their licenses.

The professional code of ethics established by the nursing profession goes beyond issues of safe practice to include standards that contribute to the quality of care of patients, their families and the community. These standards extend to issues of respect, patient advocacy and professional competence. Respecting and caring for patients regardless of age, race, ethnicity, economic status, personal attributes or nature of their health problems is a key component. There can be no prejudice against those nurses care for; all patients must receive the same standard of care. To assure this principal will be engaged, nurses are taught to evaluate themselves to ensure that they are not shortchanging any patient. If they find that their attitudes or feelings are interfering with the care they are providing, they need to take steps to remedy it.

Patient advocacy is a key component in the nurses' code of ethics. In this light, the privacy of patients must always be protected and they should be safeguarded from incompetence, unethical or illegal practices. If a nurse sees someone being given misinformation, it must be corrected and reported. Nurses cannot just close their eyes to such happenings. If a healthcare

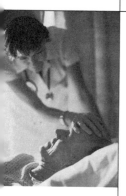

provider is too busy to properly care for a patient, it is the nurse who must intercede, even if that healthcare provider is a physician. The prime concerns for the nurse are the patients and ensuring that all of their needs are evaluated and appropriately met.

Professional nurses are also taught that their care extends to more than the patients they are serving. Patients have families who need care, comfort and understanding, and care can fail if their support systems are not recognized and included. Likewise the patient's background and culture must be taken into consideration when giving care. Recognizing the impact of illness on jobs and home life can facilitate rehabilitation and wellness.

Professional nurses need to know when to consult and with whom, when to refer a patient and how to collaborate with others about patient care. In addition, nurses must be visible members of the community to promote health. It is important to get involved by speaking to groups, initiating community programs and advocating for healthcare. These standards apply to nurses practicing in hospitals, institutions and in community settings.

Finally, a nurse's mandate includes enhancing the development of the profession itself. Nurses need to join nursing organizations, be active in them and take responsibility to help the profession have an impact on the healthcare of the nation. Are nurses more ethical than other people are? Their patients think so. A 1999 Gallup Poll Survey found that patients trust nurses more than anyone else in healthcare.[1] They are viewed as professional, dependable people, and from what I have seen and experienced, it's warranted.

Dr. Jan Towers is the Director of Health Policy at the American Academy of Nurse Practitioners in Washington, DC. She has been active in the area of health policy at the national level for over fifteen years and has served as a health policy and curriculum consultant for multiple government and private education programs and agencies. Additionally, Dr. Towers has authored numerous publications and is the founding editor of Journal of the American Academy of Nurse Practitioners.

1 The Gallup Organization. "Nurses Displace Pharmacists at Top of Expanded Honesty and Ethics Poll". 16 Nov. 1999. http://www.gallup.com/poll/releases/pr991116.asp

practice areas

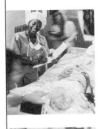

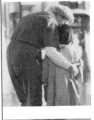

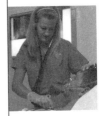

chapter one

academic nurse

A TRUE TALE

Elizabeth A. McFarlane, DNSc, RN, FAAN, remembers that her mother had always wanted to be a nurse. She recalls, too, how her mother read her books about nurses and told her stories until one day she, too, shared her mother's dream. McFarlane was able to make her dream a reality. As her career evolved she was introduced to the role of the nurse educator in an academic setting, and it fascinated her.

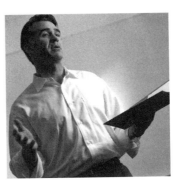

After earning a BSN from St. John College in Cleveland, Ohio in 1964, she worked at the Cleveland Clinic Hospital on a medical-surgical unit, first as a staff nurse during the day and then as an evening charge nurse. Her marriage to an officer in the United States Army began an odyssey that took her to Europe and then across the U.S., landing her in a variety of nursing jobs. When her husband's tour in Germany was interrupted with orders for Vietnam, McFarlane decided to spend the year he'd be away back in Cleveland. At the same time, the head of the nursing program at her Cleveland alma mater heard McFarlane was returning to the area and offered her a job as a senior level instructor. That position influenced her nursing career by pointing her towards academics.

Subsequent to teaching sophomore and senior nursing students at St. John's, McFarlane coordinated a Licensed Practical Nursing Program in Athens, GA, taught in an Associate Degree Program in Copperas Cove, TX, and served as Director of Staff Development at Cushing Memorial Hospital in Leavenworth, KS. In between teaching positions, she kept current in patient care by working as a staff nurse and volunteering as a Red Cross nurse in hospitals and clinics.

Those teaching opportunities McFarlane experienced convinced her that she should continue to develop her career as a nurse educator, but she realized that to guarantee future employment in academia, she would have to pursue graduate study. In 1974, when her husband's career brought him to Washington DC, McFarlane enrolled as a full-time graduate student at The

Academic Nurse Checkpoint

Do you like an educational environment?

Do you like research?

Would you be happy touching the lives of future nurses as opposed to patients in your everyday work?

If so, read on

Catholic University of America (CUA). After two years of course work she was awarded a Master of Science in Nursing (MSN) degree. Realizing that a doctorate was becoming an important credential for teaching in university settings, she extended her study at CUA to pursue a Doctor of Nursing Science (DNSc) degree. While involved in doctoral course work, she worked part-time supervising RN students enrolled in the BSN program at George Mason University in Fairfax, VA. And then, as she began work on her doctoral dissertation in 1978, she was recruited to teach full time at CUA.

A day in the life

The opportunity to work with students in the classroom as well as in the clinical area lets McFarlane have a greater influence on improving patient care than she would as a general nurse. "By teaching the principles of excellent nursing care to groups of students each year, I can make a real contribution to improving the quality of care."

Typically, McFarlane arrives at work between 7:00am and 8:00am to read and respond to e-mail. One recent weekday she attended a board meeting at a community employment training center, returned to campus to attend a curriculum meeting, met with a student, and then led a three-hour seminar focusing on measuring educational outcomes. After the class, she met and advised a doctoral student in the final stages of preparing her dissertation proposal. At 6:10pm, when she left the university, McFarlane carried home a draft of another doctoral student's dissertation to read. "A difficult aspect of my job is the need to take work home with me," McFarlane laments. "There are always classes to prepare, papers to read, and committee assignments to complete."

Teaching has solved some of her yearning to be "bedside" in the hospital, home, community centers and clinics, because she works with students in those surroundings. In an effort to bring the reality of clinical practice with teaching, McFarlane sometimes brings patients into the classroom to talk about their experiences with chronic illness and what aspects of their care were important to them.

Profiling the job

During her tenure at CUA, McFarlane has held a number of positions that have extended her faculty role. Within the School of Nursing she has served as Director of Continuing Education, director of a training grant to prepare nurse practitioners, Assistant Dean for Graduate Studies, and Associate Dean for Academic Affairs. Currently she carries a full-time teaching load, supplemented by service to the university and surrounding community.

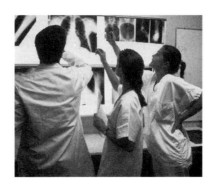

During the past two years she chaired the Academic Senate, the body that shares with the university's president responsibility for academic governing of the university. She also co-chaired the university's self-study in preparation for regional accreditation. Yet it is the interactions with students that she finds most satisfying. This semester she is teaching two graduate level courses and guiding the doctoral dissertations of eight students. One of her courses prepares graduate students for the role of nurse educator. Most recently she co-authored a book chapter on academic roles and responsibilities, and last year she presented a series of lectures on the nursing process to nurses at five different locations in Japan.

McFarlane says what is changing most about the faculty role is "the setting in which teaching and learning takes place. Over the past 10 years there has been a renewed focus on the importance of students actively participating in the teaching-learning experience." E-learning or web-based instruction has become a reality, with many nursing schools already providing online courses. While many courses will be available exclusively online, McFarlane believes that web-based instruction should be used only to supplement classroom sessions in many academic institutions. The role of the teacher, in this environment of cutting-edge technology, is frequently described as changing from the "sage on the stage" to the "guide on the side." In preparation for this role shift, faculty spend considerable time learning how to best use web-based instruction.

Regardless of the demands placed on the nurse educator, McFarlane finds the rewards plentiful. "The greatest reward," McFarlane says, "is when a student who has been having difficulty grasping a concept finally gets it!

"When you teach, you touch lives forever!"

Elizabeth A. MacFarlane, DNSc, RN, FAAN

In addition, you know you've been successful when alumnae and alumni contact you years after they have graduated to tell you how you touched their lives in a special way."

McFarlane attributes her own success as a nurse educator to the nurses in clinical practice and academia who served as role models to her. These men and women had high expectations not only of themselves, but of the nurses working with them.

STUDENT POINT OF VIEW

One of the most important things students want, McFarlane says, is for their teachers to be available to them and to encourage them. It helps if the instructors are enthusiastic about what they teach. "You can't hope to set student nurses on fire unless you radiate it yourself," she says.

>>> fast facts

What do you need?
- Knowledge of educational principles and a passion for teaching
- To be skilled in current concepts in staff education
- Three to five years of research or teaching assistance experience

What's it take?
- A current state RN license
- A BSN degree
- Sometimes a master's degree is required

Where will you practice?
- Hospitals
- Classrooms
- Research laboratories
- Higher education settings

chapter two

acute care nurse practitioner

A TRUE TALE

Like many young people, Kathy Magdic, MSN, RN, ACNP-CS, had a personal experience which would ultimately change the course of her life. When she was a small girl she contracted polio. The disease required multiple surgical procedures throughout her grade school years to allow her to walk. While in the hospital, nurses offered her comfort and friendship and talked to her about her illness. "By the time I reached high school, I had decided to be one of them," says the 49-year-old Pittsburgh native.

After graduation from high school, Magdic entered a hospital-based nursing program. Initially she wanted to work on a medical-surgical unit. There were no available positions, however, so she was forced to accept her second choice — the cardiology unit.

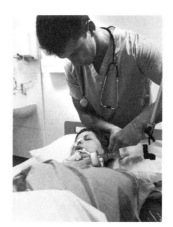

Magdic eventually pursued a BSN from Penn State University. Within a year after receiving her degree, Magdic decided she wanted to pursue a career as an advanced practice nurse. This decision led her to graduate school where she received an MSN as a Cardiopulmonary Clinical Nurse Specialist from the University of Pittsburgh School of Nursing. As a result of her experience with patients with cardiovascular disease, Magdic was recruited to help develop the cardiopulmonary subspecialty in the Acute Care Nurse Practitioner (ACNP) program at the University of Pittsburgh.

After obtaining her ACNP degree in 1995, she began working in the Cardiac Pavilion Service at the University of Pittsburgh Medical Center, an inpatient service run by a team of attending nurse practitioners, and one physician assistant. The service's average census ranges from 20–30 patients per day and includes patients diagnosed with a variety of cardiovascular diseases. In addition, patients with other medical-surgical diagnoses are admitted to this service for constant cardiac monitoring when required, because of a history of cardiac disease.

Acute Care Nurse Practitioner Checkpoint

Are you self-motivated and not afraid to ask questions?

Are you curious and interested in pathology?

Does a combination of patient care and management issues appeal to you?

If so, read on

An important component of her job includes spending time discussing the plan of care with the patient and family. "I very much enjoy this aspect of my job. Many times I am thanked by the patient and family for taking the time to listen. A few extra minutes spent with the patient can alleviate a lot of anxiety," says Magdic.

A day in the life
Today, Magdic's working day typically begins with patient rounds at 7:45am. She performs physical assessments, follows up on laboratory and diagnostic tests and collaborates with the attending physician along with the nurses and other members of the healthcare team.

When new patients are admitted, Magdic performs a physical exam, discusses the plan of care with the attending physician and writes the admission orders. Some days the service gets eight new admissions, while on other days only a few come in. Other responsibilities surrounding a patient's care are dictated by the needs of the patient. While ACNPs are trained to do a variety of procedures, there is not much opportunity for Magdic to put them into practice on the Cardiac Pavilion Service. "A constant stream of new patients are admitted every day. Just getting them medically stabilized keeps us in a state of perpetual motion," she says.

"In addition to patient contact, what I love most about my job as an ACNP is the autonomy and ability to make decisions about patient care and management issues in the field of cardiology."

The length of a patient's stay varies considerably. Those admitted for a balloon angioplasty can be discharged in as short a time as 23 hours, while patients suffering from congestive heart failure can be retained for weeks. Another part of her day includes discharging patients. This means writing the discharge orders, giving instructions to the patient and family and dictating a discharge summary of the patient's stay.

ACNPs function in a variety of settings. Many are employed by hospitals to cover inpatient services. Others are hired by physician practices where they may see patients not only in the hospital, but also in the office where the patient comes for follow-up services.

Profiling the job

In the Pittsburgh market, the pay scale for an ACNP ranges from $38,000 to $60,000 a year, which she feels "does not correspond with our training and ability." Medicare now recognizes NPs in any geographic location, but still, some private third-party providers do not routinely reimburse for services.

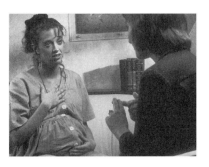

To succeed as an ACNP, Magdic says you have to be self-motivated and confident enough to ask questions. You also have to be resourceful and know who has the answers. It's good to be well-versed in your field and "to have a pocketful of reference material," she says. "You'll need it."

Not a day goes by that Magdic doesn't learn something new while practicing. There has never been a patient that she's cared for who hasn't taught her something. Often what she sees on the floor sets her off on research missions. One patient with cardiomyopathy and congestive heart failure was not a candidate for a heart transplant but was being treated with an experimental biventricular pacemaker. In this instance, she went looking for information on biventricular pacemakers and studied how pacing both ventricles reduces the risk of heart failure and ameliorates the symptoms of its onset.

Acute care nurse practitioners as a specialty will grow, she predicts, because physicians appreciate their expertise in the field and increasingly are creating positions to incorporate them in their practices. "ACNPs bring to a practice not only the medical piece, but also their nursing roots. Working in collaboration with a physician is like a good marriage — each one brings to the table something unique yet complementary. In the end, the patient wins," she adds. She considers the field of nursing one of life's nobler professions and admits she would be pleased if either of her two sons were to choose nursing as a career path. "It would mean they care about mankind," she says.

Caring for patients with heart disease for so many years has made Magdic no stranger to death. That has made her take her own mortality as well as the concept of death more in stride and, ironically, has made her more confident. But it has also intensified her feelings that our healthcare system "doesn't let people die right. We hold on to them long after they're ready to go."

PATIENT POINT OF VIEW

The 25-year-old man was diagnosed with pleurisy and pneumonia, which confined him to an acute care hospital bed. One of his lungs had filled with fluid. Coughing pushed his ribs against his lungs, causing excruciating pain. Most nights, medications and the gentle coaxing from nurses lulled him to sleep long before the expectorant kicked in. One night, however, his lungs got the better of him. Like magic, a nurse appeared at his bed and pushed against his side, keeping the inflamed lung from pressing against his ribs, preventing what would have been, the young man said later, "an unbearable agony."

>>> fast facts

What do you need?
o   Course work in:
  – Physiology
  – Pathophysiology
  – Pharmacology
  – Advanced physical assessment
  – Advanced diagnostics
  – Management
o   Over 700 clinical hours focusing on advanced physical assessment, advanced diagnostics, and advanced patient care

What's it take?
o   An active RN license
o   A master's or higher degree in nursing
o   Preparation as an adult acute care nurse practitioner

Where will you practice?
o   Critical care units
o   Other inpatient areas
o   Physician offices
o   Emergency and urgent care settings
o   Specialty outpatient clinics
o   Home care settings

cardiology nurse

A TRUE TALE

Bill Thompson, RN, BSN, CCRN, has always been fascinated by the heart. "It's one of the best understood organs in the body," he says, "yet we are still learning about it." Thompson made his decision to become a cardiology nurse in anatomy class in the first year of college, casting aside pharmacy and accounting, the other careers he'd considered.

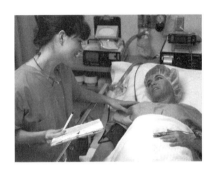

Now he works the 3:00pm to 11:00pm shift at Moses Taylor Hospital in Scranton, PA, caring for critically ill cardiac patients. Because of the high-risk nature of heart disease, Thompson usually cares for one or two patients at the most. The usual ratio is typically around eight patients to one nurse. Thompson's patients can't always talk to him because they are often sedated or on life support. But their hearts communicate with him through advanced telemetry and monitoring systems — standard equipment for this high-tech specialty. When his patients are awake, he keeps them busy with medications, pulmonary therapy, meals, and easy movement. Between tending to a patient's needs, assessing vital signs and caring for their hearts, he rarely sits down for the entire shift.

A day in the life

Thompson is on the phone at least five times a night with a cardiologist. "These physicians depend on my assessment skills. Often they make their patient's management decisions based on the urgent issues we discuss," he says.

"Some nights, though rare, are slow. That's a good time for me to teach visiting family members how to care for the patient at home. I explain how to give cardiac medications, which signs and symptoms to look out for — that is, what might signal a new heart event, and when it's imperative to get in touch with the physician."

Cardiology Nurse Checkpoint

Are you detail-oriented?

Can you handle the life and death intensity of cardiac surgery?

Does the incredible power of the human heart captivate you?

If so, read on

Four out of five patients who come in with heart failure or a heart attack survive. To relieve a life-threatening blood clot lodged in a coronary artery, surgeons often go after the clot with one of several available drugs administered as soon as possible after a heart attack, to break up the clot and get the blood flowing again. On average, patients stay in cardiac critical care after they are stabilized for three days before they're transferred to a heart monitor unit.

Profiling the job

Thompson, who says there is a higher percentage of men in cardiac nursing than in some other specialties, received a Bachelor of Science in Nursing from Thomas Jefferson University in Philadelphia in 1995 after interning at the Mayo Clinic. After graduation, the 27-year-old became a staff nurse in a Telemetry Unit for a year before moving to the cardiac intensive care unit.

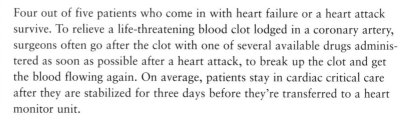

"Although there's little long-term follow-up and sustained patient contact, cardiology nursing can be very rewarding. If a patient comes in with heart failure, we're the ones who perform the magic. And we can continue to manage their conditions over time."

On the cardiac floor, he has had many heart-warming experiences. A 50-year-old woman cardiac-arrested right in front of him. In no time, Thompson had the fibrillating heart back to normal sinus rhythm.

Although Thompson is heartened by events in the cardiac unit, he expects to move on at some point. "Burn-out is a very real issue, but nursing has such a broad spectrum of specialties that would be interesting to try," he says. Oddly, patient case loads seem to be seasonal. "We get more heart attacks in winter and congestive heart failure in the spring and summer," he says. "For some reason, September through March is high season. We get a lot of very sick patients and periodically there are weeks when a lot of them, unfortunately, die."

But even that has its recompense. Early in his nursing career, Thompson was devastated when a young woman who was a patient died. "That reminded me that no life is not expendable; that there are no guarantees. I definitely take time to enjoy little things, to live my own life to the fullest."

PATIENT POINT OF VIEW
Tales From the Bedside: Comfort, No Cure

She was old, pale, and cachexic. When I walked in, Mrs. B. was lying still, tears falling from the corners of her eyes as she tried to splint the left side of her chest with her hands. Her family was around her, looking helpless as they watched her suffer.

Mrs. B. was tired beyond caring. End stage heart failure had left her with no energy to eat or move, but her mind and speech were clear. I set up the morphine pump quickly, programming the computer on it for a "bolus" (big loading dose of morphine) to be followed by a steady infusion. I punched in the "start" sequence, and watched the dose scroll by on the monitor and the piston depress the syringe. I had to make sure that the dose the pump was programmed to give correlated with the actual amount dispensed. All the while I kept up a patter, hoping to distract Mrs. B. from her pain.

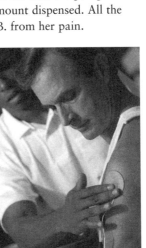

Eventually, the wrinkles on her face softened, but her hands were still pressed hard on her rib cage. I turned her on her side with her painful ribs up, making sure that her body was aligned and balanced to allow her to relax. I rubbed her head softly while explaining to the family my plan of care for the night. Then I assured them I'd be taking care of her until 7:30am. When I finished in the room, she was sleeping.

She woke in the middle of the night. I knew when she awoke because the artifact in the ECG tracing started moving irregularly. I went into her room. She looked around, frightened. When she saw me she was startled, "I dreamed I was at home," she said. I refreshed her memory and she reached for my hand as I spoke to her, gripping it with a surprising and desperate strength. I sat in the chair near her bed and looked at her. Her pain was gone, her face was relaxed, as she spoke about her family and "the good old days." Then she became very serious. "I'm scared of dying. I know

Did you know?
Women get heart attacks on average ten to 15 years later than men, but over the course of a lifetime, heart attacks become an equal-opportunity affliction.

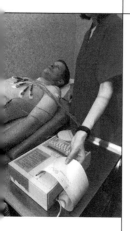

I'm getting sicker, and what will happen eventually. I pray and talk about it, and still I'm frightened." I listened and waited with her while she drifted off to sleep again, peaceful and relaxed.

I realized then that I, too, was scared. I couldn't offer her more life, couldn't fix her failing heart, couldn't make her better. All I could offer her was a massage, a clean bed, an easing of her pain, a ready ear, and an open heart. Sometimes, that's enough.

The next morning, Mrs. B awoke bright and cheerful. Her son was amazed at the difference in his mother. She took his hand gently and spoke to him in a soft voice, smiling a smile that comes from the resolution of conflict. She was happy, loving and pain-free.

That morning when I stopped in to say goodbye, she was still lively and chatty, but the light from the morning sun showed the dark, red-purple circles under her eyes. The next night my patient assignment had changed but I stuck my head in to say hello to Mrs. B. She was comatose, barely breathing, and sallow. Her children were in the room, grief-stricken over the change in their mother's condition. I hugged them and then walked around the bed, reached over the rails and stroked her head. It was warm, with the light sheen of perspiration that comes from narcotic use. Her eyes were closed, her countenance relaxed. If not for the occasional rise and fall of her chest you would think she was already gone. I muttered a small benediction, then went back to take care of my new patients.

Alwin Hawkins, RN, has been doing critical care nursing with a focus on cardiology for 15 years, and has been a registered nurse for almost 20 years. He works a 12-hour night shift in the Coronary Care Unit at Providence St. Vincent's Medical Center in Portland, Oregon.[1]

Did you know?
Approximately 250,000 people per year die of a heart attack before reaching a hospital.

fast facts

What do you need?
- A current job with experience in a cardiac care setting (eight hours per week)
- A minimum of 2,000 hours of hospital experience either in critical care or acute coronary care
- Thirty hours of continuing education applicable to cardiac rehabilitation within the past three years

What's it take?
- BSN preferred, ADN usually sufficient for entry level
- Two years of practice as a licensed RN
- Successful completion of the American Heart Association ACLS program

Where will you practice?
- Cardiac clinics
- Medical centers
- Hospitals
- Outpatient cardiac management programs
- Nursing homes

1 Alwin Hawkins. "Tales From the Bedside: Comfort, No Cure". http://viewfromtheheart.com

chapter four
chemical dependence
rehabilitation nurse

**Chemical
Dependence
Rehabilitation
Nurse
Checkpoint**

Can you be
compassionate
toward people
who are self-
destructive?

Would it give
you great
pleasure to
know you
played a role
in changing
someone's life?

Are you
interested in
helping people
get through
a mental
and physical
recovery
process?

If so, read on

A TRUE TALE

Though her younger years were not easy ones, Barbara Della always "kept her eyes on the prize." She wanted only to be a nurse and with hard work and an unwavering goal, she made it. Della, an RN with experience in neurology and med-surg, has been working at Daytop Village, a rehabilitation facility in Far Rockaway, New York, for the past twelve years. Clients stay at the residential facility for three to 18 months, so "we really get to know them," says Della. It's a voluntary program that serves people on both an "in" and "out" patient basis. Most of the treatment costs are covered by Medicaid or private insurance, but some clients self-pay. To determine if a client is suitable for residential treatment, a series of medical, legal and

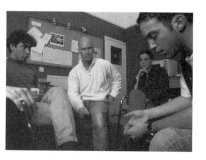

psychiatric screenings are performed. People accepted for admission are transferred to upstate New York for nine to 12 months. After that period, they return to Far Rockaway where they stay for another month to a year, depending on what's waiting for them outside. If they have marketable skills, and if they can find a job, they leave.

Della started working as a staff nurse at Daytop and eventually was promoted to nursing supervisor. Today she runs the medical department, which has a staff of nine nurses, three physicians, two nutritionists and a medical assistant. Up to 100 patients enter her unit each day, including new clients and re-entries. Some patients merely stop by for medication.

A day in the life

Della is responsible for supervising physical exams, blood work and medical screenings for all newly admitted patients. She also tends to charts and lab requisitions, participates in problematic case conferences and multidisciplinary meetings, runs a daily staff meeting, compiles budget reports and sits on various committees. And, she is on the spiritual retreat team for Daytop's HIV-positive clientele. Della estimates that eight percent of Daytop's 1,100 residents are HIV-positive.

"Addicted clients can be difficult, needy and manipulative. Some try to pull one over on us — to get out of doing something they don't want to do, by faking illness. But it's our job to be aware of things like that. The longer we work with these patients, the better we understand why they do what they do. This is very helpful for both us and them. As nurses, we're advocates for our patients. We take their complaints seriously and treat them as a nurse would treat any patient."

Profiling the job

While Della practices a variant of tough love, she feels more love than toughness for her patients. Periodically, someone will come in to thank her for sticking with him or her, for helping save his or her life when no one else thought they'd make it, she says.

"Seeing people graduate and return a year later, maybe married now, or back with their family, living as contributing members of society — that's the best thing about what I do. But unfortunately, only about half of our residents succeed." The worst thing, she concedes, "is watching the ones who don't make it and don't get the message. Some get lost in the system. Others die. This disease can be devastating."

Dependency rehabilitation is a growing specialty, especially today, as drugs are increasingly prevalent among younger people, she says. At the same time, more money is being committed to treat substance addictions, in large part, because it helps to reduce crime. Even with a current nursing shortage, her facility is fully staffed. She attributes this to the stable hours — nine to five — and weekends and holidays off. "At Daytop we have excellent benefits, too, and don't take care of bedridden people," she says. "That can be hard on nurses." What she likes best is the constant stimulation. "It's never boring here.

"One hundred percent of our patients are substance abusers. Heroin, crack, cocaine, alcohol, marijuana — any drug that's out there, our population has done it," she says.

"Seeing people graduate and return a year later, maybe married now, or back with their family, living as contributing members of society... that's the best thing about what I do."

Barbara Della, RN

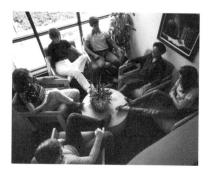

We have a variety of nursing experiences beyond treating addiction, from HIV management, to diabetes and hepatitis, plus many of the other diseases you'd see in a hospital setting."

PATIENT POINT OF VIEW

By the time patients "turn themselves in" for help, they recognize they have a problem that they have not been able to solve on their own. They seek counseling with behavioral modification techniques and hope for comfort and concern from their nurses. They do not want to be judged or belittled. These are the things that got them started on the "bad stuff." After hitting rock bottom, they begin to realize how much they require strict guidance and demarcated limits to regain their footing.

fast facts

What do you need?
- Three years of experience as an RN
- Two years of practice in rehabilitation nursing within five years of the certification exam
- Experience with a wide variety of mental health problems

What's it take?
- A current, unrestricted RN license
- A BSN from a four-year college
- Certification in addictions (CARN)

Where will you practice?
- Prevention programs
- Traditional outpatient programs
- Intensive outpatient programs
- Outpatient methadone clinics
- Detoxification centers
- Hospital based inpatient settings
- Residential treatment settings
- Mental health clinics
- Trauma centers
- Emergency rooms
- Employee assistance programs

chapter five
child psychiatry nurse

**Child Psychiatry
Nurse
Checkpoint**

Do you
see "mental"
health as equal
to physical
health?

Are you
content to be
able to help
people cope
rather than
to cure them?

Can you avoid
telling people
what to do,
but rather
point them in
the right direc-
tion?

If so, read on

A TRUE TALE

In 1985, a few months before the Challenger exploded, the 42-year-old babysitter of Donna Gaffney's three children, died of breast cancer. That same week, a dear friend of her then 9- and 12-year old sons died in a

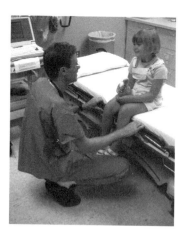

camping accident. Gaffney, who at the time was working on her doctorate in nursing science, found there were few resources to help her children deal with the emptiness in their lives resulting from the deaths of their friend and their beloved babysitter. She listened as her children expressed their sadness and learned a lot about what they needed. Then and there, Gaffney resolved to create guidelines for adults dealing with grieving children. Two years later, New American Library published her book, *The Seasons of Grief: Helping Children Grow Through Loss.*

In January, 1986, when the spacecraft carrying a beloved teacher detonated in the skies as millions of horrified school children watched on their TV screens, a producer for "Today" invited Gaffney on the show to talk about the impact on children and what families could do to get through the collective trauma. Subsequently, Gaffney's resolve to mine this field strengthened.

A day in the life

Gaffney began her career in pediatrics with a Bachelor of Science in Nursing. She spent three years in the pediatric intensive care unit at The New York Hospital, where she saw critically ill children and watched their parents and siblings deal with the crisis of hospitalization. "I realized that the psychological and emotional needs of children and families facing this crisis seemed a powerful need for me to address," says Gaffney.

So Gaffney returned to Teacher's College for a master's degree in child development and then went on to Rutgers University for an advanced practice degree in psychiatric mental health nursing. After that, the mother of three enrolled for a doctorate at the University of Pennsylvania. Upon completing her doctorate, Gaffney moved to the Columbia University School of Nursing to teach human development and child psychology, and ultimately, to head its psychiatric/mental health nursing program. In the seven years that she ran that graduate program, she privately counseled children and families in crisis — from death, divorce, illness, disasters, and accidents, to plane crashes. (She has worked with families who had children on Pan Am Flight 103, which went down over Scotland more than a decade ago). At the same time, she created community workshops for schools, corporations and groups. She recently conducted groups for third, fourth and fifth grade girls in a New York City public school. The young girls learned from literary heroines who served as positive role models in their own lives.

More recently, Gaffney has expanded her interests to the international arena, coordinating the International Trauma Studies Program at New York University. She is also involved in workshops on violence in the United States. With the New York State Division of Criminal Justice Services, she helps health providers assess and treat those sexually assaulted and abused. Her programs are offered through the Pace University Law School Women's Justice Center.

Profiling the job

With all those components of her professional life, Gaffney has no "typical day." She hasn't owned a nursing uniform since 1980. Her salary is indeterminate. Physicians refer patients to her and she refers patients to them.

Gaffney charges $1,000 per day for workshops and $80 to $100 for a 45-minute to one-hour private session. And with managed care and Medicare, she says she now gets reimbursed from several insurance companies (who often cap the number of visits patients may make), although 60 to 70 percent of her private patients still pay from their own pockets.

Gaffney believes a professional needs to create his or her own job opportunities, by getting out into the community and offering classes and workshops. "I tell my students that

"The future of mental health nursing is brilliant. With parents concerned about their children and helping them cope, these nurses are becoming more proactive. As a result, mental health treatment has become a means to take care of a family's healthcare issues," she says. "The mental health field is losing some of the stigma that previously had been attached to it."

"I pay attention to my patients' bodies, but unlike pediatric nursing I am focused first on their emotional needs. The best thing is seeing how resilient the human spirit is."

Donna Gaffney, DNSc

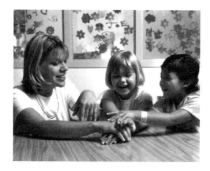

when you offer your services *pro bono,* in six months to a year you will receive offers and requests with dollar signs on them" she says. "Life and nursing are much more limited if you only sit and read want ads."

Even so, the opportunities in the field are promising. Mental illness is a critical public health problem as disabling and serious as cancer and heart disease. It is a leading cause of disability in the U.S. A U.S. Surgeon General's Report on Mental Health says:

○ Mental disorders affect one in five Americans, including children, adolescents, adults, and the elderly.

○ Stigma and its accompanying discrimination constitute the greatest barrier we face when addressing the issue of mental health. Our greatest weapon against that stigma is knowledge.

Gaffney says that there are big pluses and minuses to her specialty. "I pay attention to patients' bodies, but unlike pediatric nursing, I am focused first on the emotional needs of children. The best thing is seeing how resilient the human spirit is. People survive and thrive in the most difficult circumstances. I am their trail guide. I don't tell them what to do but point them in the right direction to explore their experiences. But the patients do all the work."

"It's incredibly challenging and rewarding to have people respond to you, to help them deal with trauma, to allow them to express their anger, fear or pain, and then to help them move to a higher level of functioning. Initially, as you work with a family or a child, it can be overwhelming or painful, but when you watch very disturbed children over time, you see how they have integrated what's happened to them into their lives and know that they will grow from it. With help, their pain is replaced by a real appreciation for life. The threads of a child's painful experience become a part of his or her own tapestry. I don't try to obliterate the pain but help those struggling to grow from it."

On the other hand, Gaffney admits, "Seeing someone angry and suffering is difficult, because I know I have to wait for them to work through their

Did you know?
Mental disorders — conditions that impair thinking, feeling, and behavior and interfere with a person's capacity to be productive and to enjoy fulfilling relationships — affect millions of Americans.

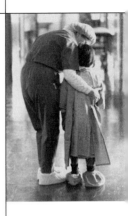

experience. There is no magic wand or instant cure. Everything takes time to heal, and that is painful." So is the realization that the issues children deal with today are more complex than they were when she was a child. "When the Columbine tragedy occurred, children across America knew about it instantly." In describing the personal effects on her own life, she says, "You really have to protect yourself, separate your work from your day-to-day life and sometimes that is not so easy. A patient often reminds you of someone in your own family." Gaffney keeps a journal to purge and explore this anxiety. She regularly talks with colleagues about cases, meditates and does yoga and always searches for balance in her life.

That might include counseling her children's friends. When her daughter went abroad for college, she urged her daughter and her daughter's friends to "call Dr. Donna" if they needed help. She celebrates when balance is restored to her patients' lives. Four years ago, she worked with a young family where the father died suddenly. The three daughters (twelve, nine, and six years old) and their mother were struggling in different ways. The youngest, for example, thought she'd done something wrong that caused her dad to die. But within five months of Gaffney's visits they were able to incorporate what had happened, to talk about it together and to plan and create a memory book. Two years later the family moved away and the mother started dating. Gaffney hears glad tidings from them at holidays.

Gaffney says the following secrets of her trade can be good indicators for this specialty:

o   You must love to listen to children

o   You have to respect children and meet them at their level

o   You must recognize that children are capable of articulating their feelings and identifying solutions to their problems

o   You have to understand that children are the experts in their own lives; the therapist merely supports and guides

Gaffney says she has learned a lot from her work. "From watching people struggle, cope and grow — you learn a great deal about yourself. You begin to understand what you need to address in your own life and why things affect you as they do. This professional specialty offers me an extraordinary opportunity to grow and it has made me a better human being."

"One patient annually calls me to announce, "I think it's time for a checkup from the neck up."

Donna Gaffney, DNSc

PATIENT POINT OF VIEW

"I think it's time for a checkup from the neck up," one patient annually calls Dr. Gaffney to announce. Most patients don't treat their mental health as conscientiously as they do their physical health. Few, for example, come in for an annual "mental" the way they do for their annual physical. Most only seek medical help in a crisis when they feel psychologically helpless or emotionally depressed. A nurse, as part of a caring medical team, can help them incorporate what's happened to them into their lives and grow from it.

>>>
fast facts

What do you need?
- Supervised clinical practice
- Specialty-focused graduate level nursing courses (or their equivalent) in physical assessment, neuroscience, and clinical psychopharmacology
- To pass a national certifying examination which must be renewed every five years

What's it take?
- To become a psychiatric-mental health clinical nurse specialist or psychiatric nurse practitioner you will need:
  - An affinity for listening to children
  - A current license as a Registered Nurse (RN)
  - A master's or doctoral degree
  - A current RN license in child psychiatry

Where will you practice?
- Various inpatient and outpatient settings
- Specific hospitals
- Community-based or home care programs
- Local, state, and federal mental health agencies
- Self-employment

Other opportunities
- Utilization Review Nurse for a managed care company
- Patient Educator
- Risk Manager
- Chief Quality Officer
- Marketing and Development Specialist
- Corporate Manager or Executive

critical care nurse

A TRUE TALE

When Katie Green, RN, BSN, was a biology and chemistry major in Tallahassee, Florida, she had every intention of going to medical school. But one summer during college she shadowed a physician and found herself enthralled with the nursing staff and what they did. "He dealt with charts and they dealt with patients," she said.

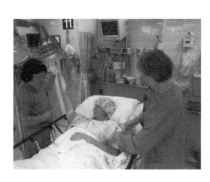

**Critical Care
Nurse
Checkpoint**

Do you have an affinity for high-tech equipment?

Will you be able to handle "losing" patients and dealing with the intense scenarios of care?

Are you prepared to put in long hours and weekends?

If so, read on

At the end of her senior year in nursing school in 1997, after a four-hour interview, recruiters from the prestigious Florida Hospital in Orlando invited Green — who was then the only one in her class to receive this invitation — to join their hospital. "I wasn't sure what I wanted to do because a million different areas intrigued me," says the 24-year-old. "But I was offered this selective prized position and took it."

Green says critical care nursing is much more focused than general nursing. "You have a few patients who are yours for at least two or three days and you become closely involved with them and their families. I learned that critical care nurses essentially run these units. When we come to work here, we have to think like the physicians — because sometimes things for our critically ill patients can turn in a second, and we've got to be prepared for that."

A day in the life

Green starts her shift assessing the three or four patients in her charge who've undergone respiratory failure, angioplasty or open heart surgery. Her principal job is to monitor vital signs and ensure the patient's medications are administered as required. She checks that the patient's IV is dispensing the drug or fluid in the correct quantity. "The biggest problems can come from miscalculating the rate of drug delivery," she says. "We use very powerful drugs in very minute amounts to manage the critically ill. Precision is of utmost importance."

The technology is very futuristic. Special computerized beds automatically weigh patients and even rotate them, and improved machinery and medicines keep pace with providing immediate output. Even a CAT scan, that used to take ten minutes, now images the patient in much less time. Green says that the upside to advanced technology is seeing the scope of its application for her various patients. But, the downside, she adds, is learning how to use it. "We have in-service classes that teach us the ins and outs, so that helps substantially."

Profiling the job

The best thing about critical care nursing is the one-on-one involvement with patients, says Green. "You have time to get to know them." In contrast, nurses on the medical-surgical floors have 10 patients and don't really know them at all, she says. A self-described "big study bug," Green says she often goes home to read about her patients' diseases. She also finds it gratifying to watch their dramatic improvement. "We see them at their sickest — and watch them recover."

The worst thing about critical care nursing — apart from a nurse shortage, which resulted in the "scary and dangerous situation" of once handling five patients — is the very same attachment that develops because of the intimate situation. "I get very attached to patients, when someone dies — and unfortunately they do — it takes me a while to get over it," Green admits.

Critical care nurses' shifts in the ICU are generally short-lived. Long hours and working weekends on top of stress generally means a quick turnaround. "It's usually just a few years before most of us move on to something easier," says Green, "but there are some nurses who make critical care a life-long career." She anticipates that she will be one to move on eventually, but doesn't feel the pull yet. Not when there is so much to learn and experience. Her most memorable lesson happened the first time she did CPR on a human rather than on a dummy. Summoned by a critical care code, Green rushed to the bed of an 80-year-old woman who'd had a heart attack, and tried to revive her. "I could feel all her ribs crack under my palms," Green recalls.

Despite the reassurance from her colleagues that this happens often with older women, the episode kept Green awake all night. But when she returned to the hospital for her next shift and saw that the woman was alive and awake, she heaved a sigh of relief.

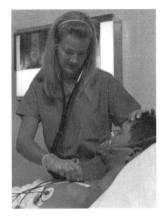

PATIENT POINT OF VIEW

In addition to being very high-tech, the ICU is fast-paced and intense. Patients' lives are constantly on the line. The nurse is the main patient care contact, collecting data and analyzing it to help make a diagnosis. But it's the behind-the-scenes activities that patients do not know much about that matter most. It is the critical care nurse who identifies an anticipated outcome, develops a plan of care and implements interventions to evaluate progress. He or she collaborates with the team, consisting of patient, family and healthcare providers, to provide patient care in a healing, humane and caring environment.

Did you know?
Critical care nursing has been around for as long as there have been critically ill patients, but didn't emerge as an organized specialty until about 1969, after ICUs were established for critically ill cardiovascular patients.

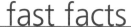

fast facts

What do you need?
- Knowledge of the physiology and management of patients who are hemodynamically monitored or on ventilators
- Experience with technology that monitors or maintains the life functions of patients
- Contribution of 1,750 or more hours caring for critically ill patients before you can take the CCRN exam

What's it take?
- A current license as a Registered Nurse
- BSN preferred, ADN usually sufficient for entry level
- State certification in critical care

Where will you practice?
- Emergency departments
- Post-anesthesia recovery units
- Medical transport services
- Step-down unit, telemetry units
- Progressive care units
- Cardiac catheterization laboratories
- Interventional radiology departments
- Clinics
- Burn units
- Pediatric intensive care units
- Neonatal intensive care units

emergency room nurse

A TRUE TALE

Kimberley Thomas, RN, fell for the emergency room (ER) while still in nursing school at Florida State University, where she earned a Bachelor of Science degree in Nursing. There, she witnessed an ER that was very fast-paced, leaving no time for boredom. And the daily work was never routine.

"Every day I learned something new. The team of nurses, physicians and other professionals rocketed from a heart attack patient to a gunshot wound, to a baby with acute asthma to a man with a fish hook in his cheek. You run the gamut from the mildest to the most severe situations and you never know what to expect."

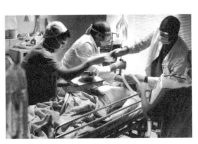

Emergency Room Nurse Checkpoint

Are you comfortable racing from one task to another?

Can you make decisions in a heartbeat?

Can you deal with the sadness of death and move on?

If so, read on

After graduating, Thomas moved to Atlanta and went to work in the ER at The Grady Memorial Hospital, a "level one" trauma center. Here she found yet another fast-paced ER environment that fueled her interest even more. "Other hospitals could divert patients but we had to maintain 24-hour availability. As a level one, we could not close our doors to an emergency — no matter how busy we were. But triaging our patients — from the sickest to the less sick — was part of the job and part of the excitement of a busy ER."

A day in the life

At The Grady Memorial Hospital, Thomas began her day at 7:00pm. Upon arrival, she received a report from the nurse who had her assignment during the day. But because more staff worked days (enabling them to divvy up the patient load), Thomas would typically have more patients to care for than the nurse before her.

First, she made fast rounds, introducing herself to each patient, making sure to ask if they were in any major pain. Then she checked their vital signs, temperature, pulse, respiratory rate and blood pressure. She made sure their charts were up to date and that they had their medicine and meals. Often she had to chase down a bed if the patient needed to be transferred to the regular nursing floor. Although these tasks sound routine, they were twice as hard because Thomas was so often interrupted by a new trauma coming in. The trick was to move fast.

When an acute trauma is on the way, the ambulance team usually calls ahead to the triage nurse (a specialized ER nurse superior who decides on patient priorities and resources) to report on their patient. The team would swing into action by putting on trauma gear, preparing all the stabilizing instruments and making sure everything they needed was there to stabilize the incoming patient as quickly as possible.

After 14 months in this position, Thomas transferred to a smaller hospital, Crawford Long, to work in their neurosurgical intensive care unit. Soon after, her desire to be back in the high pressure environment of the ER brought her to a new opportunity: working for an agency. In this capacity, Thomas is a "traveler," working temporary stints at understaffed ERs across the country. Her first assignment was in the ER at Albert Einstein Hospital in the Bronx, New York. Thomas is now working in an ER in a hospital in Philadelphia for two years. "Who knows what ER lies ahead. Wherever I go, I can be sure my life will be filled with new and exciting challenges. This is what I've grown to love."

Profiling the job

Among the many advantages of working for an agency is higher pay, which is often double that of a staff nurse. The flexibility is there, too. Thomas decides when she'll work. If she wants weekends or holidays off, she gets them. Most staff nurses are required to work three to five holidays a year; Thomas can work or not — it's up to her. But like any other nursing position there are downsides to ER work. The very nature of the work has its stresses and demands. "Sometimes you don't eat or sit down all night," says Thomas, who doubts she will stay in the ER for many more years. She can clearly remember the night that a two-year-old had been brought in from drowning and a four-year-old had been hit by

> Every day something exhilarating happens. Asthmatic patients come into the ER in distress; you give respiratory medication and they breathe again. A pregnant woman comes in with problems and leaves with a healthy baby. There's a lot of glamour and hype around an ER, but despite the adrenaline-pumping action and non-stop activity, it is still an arena for small ministrations and tender acts of mercy as well.

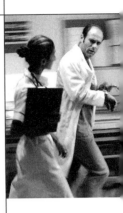

a car. "Both were pulse-less and not breathing. We got them both back — but it was touch and go there for a while," she says.

A bonus to her current position working in Philadelphia is that the hospital serves a small community, enabling Thomas to get to know the families and, on occasion, see them around town. Also, working with the same physicians every day, getting to know them and eventually earning their trust are other benefits she cites.

Thomas says there are some tricks to turn this world of total chaos into a negotiable labyrinth. For example, as a first step, she always tells patients her name. "Because we're so busy you can easily forget to be a human being," she says, "but making such a simple gesture as introducing yourself seems to put them at ease and afford a fast connection." On her first day in the ER, her preceptor cautioned her that the most important skill she'd need was to prioritize. "Follow your ABCs, she told me: airways, breathing, circulation. Then go with your instincts." Thomas adds, "not second-guessing myself has saved my patients and me many times." In one circumstance, a wizened 80-year-old man admitted to feeling "weird sensations" but urged the ER crew not to bother with him. "Something told me he was in real distress," says Thomas. After persistent urging she convinced him to let her do some quick tests. "He was in heart block, which could have killed him. And he was not the first ER patient who tried to talk me out of treatment. In fact, one patient got off his stretcher and started jogging in an attempt to prove he was healthy. He wasn't."

Thomas also jogs. "I run to get rid of stress" she says. She also vents by getting together with friends and talking things over with peers. Once when a small child was hit by a car, the team worked feverishly for 45 minutes to stabilize the very ill little boy. "After he was gone, half of us started crying," she recalled. "We know we did the best we could, and we've got to be happy with that."

Something else Thomas has learned working in the ER: "Seeing a child who has been shot puts things in perspective and reminds us how fragile and precious life really is. Now I know, really know, that in a matter of seconds, something could happen to radically change anyone's life."

"It's hard to see what we see and not absorb the sadness. But in order to continue to save the lives of others, I've learned that I have to think of myself too."

PATIENT POINT OF VIEW

To most Americans, the ER is a giant portal, the first line of health care treatment. An estimated 95 million Americans visited an emergency room last year. Millions more tune in to the popular television show "ER". That show has sparked great interest in the high-octane world of emergency medicine — a world that varies greatly, with every manner of injury and illness, from an earache to an aneurysm.

fast facts

"You've heard the term adrenaline junkie. If you don't have that in you, you don't last in here."

Randy Endsley, RN, Christus Spohn Hospital Memorial Emergency Room, Texas

What do you need?
- Skills in the fields of Advanced Cardiac Life Support, Trauma Nursing, Pediatric Emergency Nursing and Basic Cardiac Life Support
- Collaborative practice or supervision by a physician
- Emergency Nursing Association membership

What's it take?
- BSN preferred, ADN usually sufficient for entry level
- A current license as a Registered Nurse (RN)
- Certification pertinent to specific skills and abilities of practice

Where will you practice?
- Hospitals
- Clinics
- Health centers
- Private practices

flight trauma nurse

A TRUE TALE

In the 1970s, Ron Martin, RN, as a member of the Marine Corps in Vietnam, flew helicopters and fell in love with them. After his discharge he spent time as a fireman in San Diego, but was sorely frustrated that he couldn't do anything to help the victims except comfort them.

Prompted by this desire to help, at the age of 25 he went back to school with the goal of becoming a flight nurse, combining his interest in healing with his passion for flying.

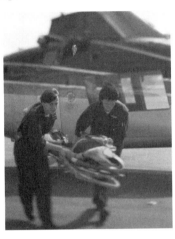

After two years at Fresno City College and armed with an associate's degree, Martin began making the rounds of nearby emergency rooms (ERs). He worked at Valley Children's Hospital, St. Agnes Hospital and University Medical Center, among others, before landing at Memorial Medical Center in Modesto, California in 1989.

Medical flights are generally dual in nature. Helicopters fly to designated spots to pick up victims of acute trauma who need transport to a large medical center. Or, they may take a critically ill patient, unable to travel by ambulance, to a hospital better equipped to handle the patient's needs.

A flight trauma nurse specializes in providing urgent and emergency care to patients during airborne transport. Flight programs vary throughout the country, but usually a paramedic and nurse go "on scene" together. Two-thirds of the requests are for "scene calls," and the remainder are inter-facility hospital transports. Martin, along with the other flight nurses and paramedics in his unit, works 12-hour shifts, rotating between days and nights. Roughly 300 transport requests, mainly from remote areas, come in each month from emergency dispatchers, police, fire departments, ski patrol or other rescue organizations. His unit transports an average of three patients a day. "Sometimes we have no calls all day and other times we have eight a shift," he says. Summer is peak season. School's out and people are more active, so there are more recreation accidents. Fog, which is a big problem in the San Joaquin Valley, is the only local weather condition that restricts

Do you want a strong background in emergency nursing?

Do you have a strong stomach for horrific scenes?

Are you comfortable flying in a helicopter?

If so, read on

response by flight. In those cases, calls are referred to ground transport ambulances. However, in other locations, weather conditions can make flight very difficult.

A day in the life

Martin and his paramedic partner are stationed close to the helipad. When they're not busy, he assists in the ER. But he's ready to run at a moment's notice when he gets paged. Usually, medical helicopters must be airborne within six minutes of receiving a call, though the average response time is closer to four minutes. During the two to three minutes it takes for the turbines to warm up, the team tracks a flight path. A medical flight helicopter is stocked with the same equipment that's standard in ambulances, plus extra medications and equipment necessary to perform some invasive procedures, should the need arise.

Flight nursing is different from general nursing because the resources are limited to what can fit into a helicopter and what can be done within the confines of such a small space. There is room for only the patient, pilot, paramedic and nurse.

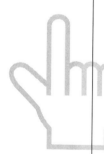

"I knew he was dying, but we had to intubate him so he could breathe. We tried to keep him comfortable and sedated. Just before we intubated him, I asked him if he wanted to say anything; I thought that might be the last words he'd ever say. He told me to tell his family he loved them."

"When a call comes in, we take off and often don't know what we'll find until we land the helicopter. It could be a two-day-old neonate with a congenital heart problem, a teenager with a gun shot wound or a motorist with a heart attack. "We never know for sure and that makes it hard for us to anticipate," he says.

In-flight medical treatment of trauma victims en route to hospitals was first used in Vietnam. Medi-Flight of Northern California was initiated in 1978 and is the oldest air ambulance in California. Memorial's flight program has saved countless lives.

Even with reduced reimbursement, there are many more air ambulance programs emerging across the country, and competition to become a flight nurse is tough. "Each month our call volume goes up," he says, "fueled by organ transplants, higher patient acuity, and the technical ability to re-implant amputations. Drugs, alcohol, crime, violence and carelessness all contribute heavily to trauma," he says.

Profiling the job

In the last 10 years in the program, Martin figures he's made over 1,000 flights. The first one though is still vivid in his mind: a truck had struck a nearly empty school bus head-on. The helicopter landed a quarter of a

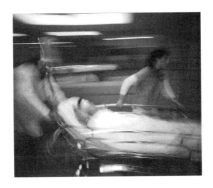

mile from the scene. In the dark, Martin ran down the road to where the victim was and brought him immediately to the helicopter. The helpers tried to load the boy into the helicopter but Martin insisted that they wait until he could assess him first on the ground — before noise of the rotor blades would drown out the sounds of the boy's vital signs.

Once airborne, Martin and his partner wear helmets and communicate with each other over the engine noise through an intercom. While still in the air, they contact the hospital to which they are heading. Emergency room nurses and physicians there are in constant contact until the patient is brought through the door. Generally, a team is dispatched to a scene and returns to base within an hour. Trauma patients must be airlifted to the nearest appropriate trauma center with a helipad. Inter-hospital patients can be transported to any tertiary hospital where necessary services can be provided. When they're brought to Memorial, Martin goes into the ER with the patient to report what he saw, how he treated it and to assist with resuscitation. He tries to follow up with his patients throughout their hospital stay.

Just as in every practice setting, sometimes the care is for naught. "The helicopter isn't called unless there's critical need," says the 52-year-old Martin. One such "need" was to attend to a man who'd caught on fire while fueling his car. When Martin arrived, the patient had third degree burns on 100 percent of his body. But because of the shock and extensive damage to nerves and tissue, he wasn't in any pain. When Martin called the hospital later, he learned that, despite everyone's best efforts, the man had died that night. "We can always do something, but that won't necessarily stave off a bad outcome," he says.

"For many people, flight trauma nursing is a lifelong goal. So once you make it there you tend to stay. There's low turnover."

Ron Martin, RN

Once he picked up a nurse co-worker in cardiac arrest but didn't recognize her until they got to hospital. "People don't look the same when they're critically ill or injured, and I think the blocking mechanism kicked in," he says. Such anguish takes its toll. "It affects your body, mind and spirit," Martin admits. As with all practitioners, Martin has learned to deal with the emotionality and stress of his work. "If we got caught up in the emotion of the family, we'd be ineffective at our jobs. Staying focused on the situation at hand requires a high degree of objectivity, emotional detachment, and concentration." To relieve job stress, Martin and his wife, who is the charge nurse of Memorial's intensive care unit, do yoga, meditation, massage, and ride their Harley Davidson motorcycles into the hills.

There are occasional miraculous outcomes. For example, Martin recalls the case of a star volleyball player and homecoming queen of a local high school who sustained major head and internal injuries and went into a coma as a result of a serious car crash. When Martin flew her in, the neurosurgeon predicted that she'd never regain consciousness. "The only thing I can say is that the strength, love and faith of her family intervened, and six weeks later she woke up," he said. She has since recovered completely and is leading a normal life.

Such stress-relievers and occasional miracles have been bandages. "We're called upon only in life-threatening situations and see the most gruesome things, horrible beyond description," he says. "Factoring in Vietnam, the body count I've seen is innumerable. And while all this tragedy has given me greater insight and inner strength, after 26 years of doing this, I'm now going back to school to become a holistic health practitioner so I can open my own business and treat the whole person. I want to see people in a different setting than the worst day of their lives."

PATIENT POINT OF VIEW
While an estimated 95 million Americans visited an emergency room last year, very few arrived by helicopter. This portable emergency room is staffed by a nurse/paramedic team that has seen it all — from difficult births to amputations, from floods to fires. Their highly intuitive judgment and diagnostic skills, coupled with fast and decisive stabilizing actions, are often what save a patient's life.

fast facts

What do you need?
- Two+ years critical care or ER experience
- Experience in Advanced Cardiac Life Support (ACLS)
- Experience in Pediatric Advanced Life Support (PALS)
- Experience in Neonatal Advanced Life Support (NALS)
- Completion of a trauma nurse core curriculum
- Completion of a flight nurse advanced trauma course

What's it take?
- License as a Certified Flight Registered Nurse (CFRN)
- License as a Certified Emergency Nurse (CEN)
- License as a Certified Critical Care Nurse (CCRN)
- A current license as a Registered Nurse (RN)

Where will you practice?
- Intensive care units
- Critical care units
- Hospitals
- Health clinics
- Air ambulance companies
- Emergency transport facilities

chapter nine
forensic nurse

Forensic Nurse Checkpoint

Do you like detective work?

Would you enjoy giving emotional support as well as physical aid to the victims of violent crimes?

Are you comfortable dealing with law enforce-ment agents?

If so, read on

A TRUE TALE

Marie Ann Marino, EdD, RN, PNP, has more advanced degrees than many physicians. The Long Island, New York native started with a BSN in 1985 and has added a doctorate of education from Teachers College at Columbia University and a post doctorate in family violence.

Marino's interest in forensic medicine surfaced while she was performing her clinical baccalaureate in pediatrics at an urban hospital in a low socio-economic community. "I fell in love with all the children but seemed to connect most, for some reason, with those who'd been abused," she says. "I saw how helpless they were; that they needed a warm shoulder to cry on and arms to just hug them. But more importantly, they required an advocate, someone who could stand up for them — especially because they could not."

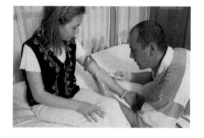

Immediately after securing her BSN, Marino went directly to work on the medical-surgical floor of Stony Brook, in New York. She expected to move into general pediatrics and figured that learning how to manage a large number of patients with different degrees of problems would be useful for this transition. But nine months later, when she requested to transfer, the only position available was in the intensive care unit (ICU).

There, she found her medical-surgical experience had molded her in unex-pected ways. "It helped me deal with families, to prioritize, and be a team player," she says. In her five years in the ICU, she attended to many children from other countries who came to the hospital to undergo surgery, some without any immediate family members for support.

Profiling the job

Forensic medicine is the science concerned with relations between medicine and the law. Forensic nurses are known for investigating deaths but Marino deals exclusively with live victims of abuse. Like other forensic nurses in other sub-specialties, she collaborates with experts in sociology, psychology, social work, political science, medicine, law enforcement, and the judicial system. In addition to domestic violence and sexual assault, forensic nurses deal with a myriad of cases ranging from food and drug tampering, non-medically supervised abortions, inappropriate medication administration, traumatic injuries, and suicide.

In 1991, Marino moved to Nassau County Medical Center as a nurse practitioner in charge of coordinating the child abuse center. Along with a team of physicians, she was responsible for evaluating all suspected child abuse cases in the clinic, emergency room, ICU, burn unit and pediatric wards. "Approximately 20 children a week gave us cause for suspicion," she notes. "The first thing we do is look and listen," she says. "You assess what the child looks like and what he or she tells you. You listen to how the parent explains the child's bruises and decide if that story matches with the child's injuries. It's putting the pieces of a puzzle together." She estimates that between 75 to 85 percent of the cases are "real."

When Marino confirms an abuse diagnosis, she refers the victim to Child Protective Services (CPS). CPS does a full investigation, which includes police involvement. When necessary, children will be hospitalized or referred to therapy, or both. Sometimes they are put in foster care. Marino often sees the children again in court, where she is called upon to testify regarding their cases.

Three years ago Marino moved to Suffolk County as the forensic medical examiner of sexually abused children. There, she operates interchangeably with the physicians and has an RN as her assistant. Her patients range in age up to 17 years. But she has also seen babies as young as three months old — a harrowing sight under any circumstance.

In areas of the country not served by a medical examiner or forensic physician, the forensic nurse may be brought in by various legal agencies to consult in cases of child abuse, sexual assault and suspicious deaths.

The criteria that set off warning flags that a child has been abused are known to everyone who works with such children. If the injuries are on the knees and elbows they're considered routine, but a bruise on the middle of the face, for example, is deemed suspicious. "Children don't usually fall flat

Did you know?
The theoretical model of forensic nursing evolved from the role of police surgeon or police medical officer in the United Kingdom and various European countries.[1]

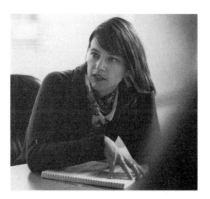

on their faces," she says. Bruises on the buttocks and thighs also are suspect. Marino has learned to gauge the age of the injury by the stage of healing. She then compares it to the parent's story of what happened to the child, and when. It's very important to do an in-depth interview with the parents. To gain access to the vulnerable population she examines, Marino says she has to rely on the parents, and so she takes care not to alienate them or make them feel intimidated. She avoids using medical terminology that might scare or confuse them. "Do that and you won't see the child again," she says. Marino estimates that her agency sees only "the tip of the iceberg," about ten percent of the area's sexually abused children.

"Contrary to some stereotypical popular misconceptions, child abuse is not primarily inflicted on poor children," says Marino. "It's a myth that it's all one race or class. Child abuse spans all types."

Despite the dark clouds, there are silver linings to her job. "Getting children out of situations where they have no power is a blessing," says Marino. And the spillover into her own life has been profound. "This has taught me how fragile children really are and how important it is to surround them with people who will guarantee their welfare."

PATIENT POINT OF VIEW

They call him Baby Georgia. He is the ten-month old boy in the emergency room who was the subject of a protective investigation. The physical injuries on his body were a road map to the suffering he had been forced to endure since he came into the world. This is the only life he knows, though. No matter how cruel it is, when he sees her, he still lifts his arms and reaches towards his mother.

"Getting children out of situations where they have no power is a blessing."

Marie Ann Marino, EdD, RN, PNP

fast facts

What do you need?
- A willingness to work with all extremes of human behavior
- A psychiatric background is helpful
- Investigative and counseling skills

What's it take?
- A current license as a Registered Nurse (RN)
- BSN preferred, ADN usually sufficient for entry level
- Master's degree may be required
- Certification may be required for Sexual Assault Nursing Examination (SANE), forensic pediatric/geriatric nurse

Where will you practice?
- Acute healthcare facilities
- Correctional institutions
- County prosecutor and coroner's office
- Medical examiner's office
- Insurance companies
- Psychiatric facilities

Forensic Nursing Careers
- Sexual Assault Nurse Examiner (SANE)
- Nurse coroner
- Nurse investigator
- Correctional nurse
- Forensic psychiatric nurse
- Pediatric/geriatric nurse educator
- Researcher
- Consultant

Did you know?
Trauma associated with violence is the leading killer of young Americans between one and 44 years of age.

1 Lynch, Virginia. "A New Perspective in the Management of Crime Victims from Trauma to Trial".
 http://www.forensicnurse.org/resource/lynch.htm

chapter ten
geriatric nurse

Geriatric Nurse Checkpoint

Do you have a desire to help people enjoy their final years?

Do you feel a connection to the elderly?

Do you see older adults as survivors and not victims?

If so, read on

A TRUE TALE

Karen Desjardins' grandmother is the reason she learned the value of older people in our society. "Though widowed for years, she remained a committed and vital teacher in downtown Chicago, no easy task for a woman her age," says the 47-year-old registered nurse and assistant professor of clinical nursing at Columbia University School of Nursing, who, for the last year, has been

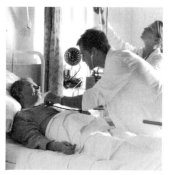

the director of the geriatric nurse practitioner program there. "Perhaps she is why I became a clinical specialist in gerontological nursing."

She adds, "I've always enjoyed working with older people. It lets me focus on the whole process of aging, as well as on biological disease. It's an added dimension as far as I'm concerned."

A day in the life

In addition to heading the gerontological nurse practitioner program at Columbia, Desjardins sees patients with dementia at its Neurological Institute. In evaluating the older adult, Desjardins assesses mental status, functional status, financial status, patient values and social support. She looks at a patient's nutrition, pain level and physical functionality as well. "You think about the personal needs of your patients. Are they eating well? Are they getting out? Do they have decent social support? Even the smallest things count. Things such as the phones being in a place where they can easily reach them in their homes. Are there scatter rugs that might pose a hazard for those using walkers?"

The well-known activist Maggie Kuhn once said, "The first myth is that old age is a disease. So you lie about your age. We'll it's not a disease, it's a triumph. You've survived failure, disappointment, sickness, loss and you're still here."

Profiling the job

Many older people feel invisible and undervalued in a society that idolizes youth. Nurses who specialize in the geriatric and the gerontological arena are a breed apart, seeing wrinkles as a testament to experience and sensing wisdom where others see decay. By and large, they're interested not only in getting the elderly back on their feet, but in having their patients enjoy what those feet represent — mobility and freedom. They're interested in wellness of mind and body and care for the whole person — which in most older people includes at least one chronic condition. While in better health than their predecessors, today's older people require more medical care than the general population, mostly because they're living longer. The 12.8 percent of America's population 65 and over account for more than 60 percent of ambulatory adult primary visits, 80 percent of home care visits, 85 percent of nursing home residents and 48 percent of hospital patients.[1]

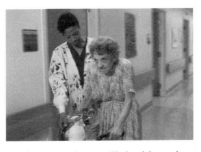

Desjardins sees her role as promoting a high level of wellness and maintaining functionality among her patient population. In addition, she acts as their public relations representative. Her goal is to foster a good healthy philosophy on aging that focuses on hope, pride and integrity. People 65 and older account for nearly 13 percent of the population. Within a few years those numbers will double and the need for geriatric and gerontological nurses will balloon accordingly, she says.

Specifically, the ailments that most frequently affect this population are cancer, arthritis, hypertension, heart disease and diabetes. "Certainly, being around aging people makes me think about my own aging — and possible morbidity associated with it. But my job has reinforced what I learned as a young girl — to have a really healthy philosophy about aging. My patients regularly teach me a lesson about dealing with what life throws at you. They're inspiring heroes."

Did you know?
In 2000, one in eight Americans was 65 or older.

By 2030, one in five Americans will be 65 or older.

Since 1970, the number of "older old" (those 85+) has more than tripled.

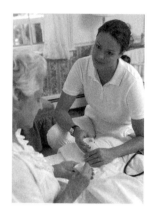

PATIENT POINT OF VIEW

The woman had Alzheimer's. She and her husband were living in a nursing home. Without fail, each day her husband visited to read aloud the words that she had recorded in her journal through the years. The nurses on the unit enjoyed watching them smile and share their memories. But one day the husband came to greet her and received a blank and unknowing stare. She didn't realize who he was. The nurse entered the room to prompt him to try again tomorrow. When he left, the woman spoke and questioned the nurse as to who the stranger at her bedside was. In a soft and caring voice the nurse explained that he was someone who enjoyed her company.

fast facts

What do you need?
- Clinical specialists must have any of the following:
  - 800 hours (post-master's) of direct patient care
  - 800 hours (post-master's) of clinical management in gerontological nursing in the past 24 months
- Consultants, researchers, educators, and administrators must have either of the following:
  - 400 hours (post-master's) of direct patient care
  - 400 hours (post-master's) of clinical management in gerontological nursing in the past 24 months
- Twelve months of practice following completion of a master's degree

What's it take?
- A current license as a Registered Nurse (RN)
- BSN preferred, ADN usually sufficient for entry level

Where will you practice?
- Hospitals
- Nursing homes
- Neighborhood clinics
- Home care
- Senior centers
- Community wellness programs

1 Roback, Lisa. "Nursing Hands. Your Nursing Career in Graying America".
http://nursinghands.com/static/careinthe.html

chapter eleven
home care nurse

Home Care Nurse Checkpoint

Would you prefer to work outside of a centralized building, and do you enjoy driving daily?

Do you like going into people's homes — even if you don't speak their language or know their culture?

Would you prefer the autonomy of being an independent health provider working alone?

If so, read on

A TRUE TALE

The reason home care nursing appealed to Judy Flynn, RN, was because she loved the one-to-one rapport with patients and the great variety they presented to her each day. "You get to know people well when you're working in their homes — sometimes you meet the family." After she graduated 30 years ago from St. Michael's Nursing School in Newark, New Jersey, Flynn

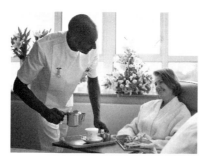

worked as a hospital nurse for seven years. She then took a certification exam which would license her to work for agencies handling health-care delivery in private homes, nursing homes, and rehabilitation centers. After passing the test, Flynn applied for a home care job with an agency serving an area not far from where she grew up.

A day in the life

Most days, the 50-year-old listens to light FM music and the news while covering around 60 miles on her daily routine of six to eight patients. Typically, she'll roll into her first driveway around 8:30am. But the status of her patients dictates when her day starts. "Sometimes I'm there earlier to check the blood sugar levels of a new patient who is diabetic, for example."

One day's agenda brings her to a patient with a leaking Foley catheter, then to draw blood from a bed-bound patient on insulin. Another patient that she has been monitoring has hypertension. Patients are responsible for their own medicine, but Flynn makes sure that the prescription has been properly stored and confirms how patients take them.

Flynn treasures the autonomy of her specialty, especially the fact that she sees patients on a one-to-one basis and in their own homes rather than in a hospital setting. "It helps you to see them as real people."

Another patient is recovering from open-heart surgery and still another from a hip replacement. In the first case, after checking vital signs, confirming medications and assessing the patient's overall status, she attends to his incision and diet. In the second, she's concerned about physical therapy and home safety and decides to call in a social worker. On one stop, she administers an injectable drug to a multiple sclerosis patient who cannot do it for herself. On another, she consults with the family of a stomach cancer patient after attending to the patient's hydration and pain control. Flynn talks to the physician if a problem arises that she cannot handle or if there's a condition that she feels he or she should know about. Many patients she'll see daily for two to three weeks before they "graduate." Older patients who often have more problems often stay on her docket for a longer time. Flynn, who has worked for a home care agency for the past 11 years, travels with a beeper that she checks consistently between home visits. Her week is never routine. "Each day is so varied," she says.

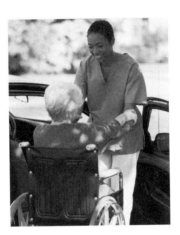

Patients welcome her visits and try to make her feel like a guest. Flynn appreciates their hospitality but also keeps things on a professional level. "It seems to work better for us all," she says.

Profiling the job

The most tedious aspect of the job is the paperwork. Flynn adheres to Medicare guidelines, which means completing 18–22 pages to "open a patient." Each visit results in at least one additional sheet. For every colleague she calls (usually two to three per patient visit) she has to write a case conference. Medicare pays the agency, which in turn pays her. Flynn says she earns just about what she would make at a hospital. But other aspects of "pay" are more intangible. "Patients often write something complimentary about me to the office and some actually joyfully wait for me to arrive," she says. Although she works in poor and what some may consider unsafe neighborhoods, she enjoys her visits. People see her blue and white or navy uniform, medical bag and name tag and usually call out friendly greetings.

"This specialty offers a view of life that encompasses patient, family and community in the broader societal context. That's where nursing started, and for all the evolution that has occurred in the delivery of healthcare, it remains the heart and soul of nursing."

Sue Thomas Hegyvary, PhD, RN, FANN, University of Washington School of Nursing

Did you know?
A century ago, virtually all medical and nursing care was provided in people's homes.

PATIENT POINT OF VIEW

Personal relationships are an essential part of every nurse-patient interaction. But to the home care patient, they are probably even more critical. For those confined at home, the visiting nurse can often be the sole contact with the outside world. The home care nurse is often far more than a healthcare provider. He or she might quickly become a friend, a bearer of news, a conversationalist or perhaps even a card partner. The point is that the patient sees his or her home care nurse as a medical professional and a visitor, a friend and an advocate. Home care nurses need a bedside manner and an understanding of the needs of the patients, who may often feel lonely and vulnerable.

fast facts

What do you need?
- A working knowledge of relevant medical technologies and care techniques
- A certificate of health, including current immunization status
- Personal malpractice insurance coverage

What's it take?
- BSN preferred, ADN usually sufficient for entry level
- A current license as a Registered Nurse (RN)
- Certification in cardiopulmonary resuscitation

Where will you practice?
- Home health agencies
- Hospices
- Homemaker and home care aide (HCA) agencies
- Staffing and private-duty agencies
- Companies specializing in medical equipment and supplies, pharmaceuticals, and drug infusion therapy

industry nurse

A TRUE TALE

In the summer of 1988 Jane Newman, RN, MPH, after graduating from the Yale School of Medicine with a Master's in Public Health, joined Pfizer to do policy analysis in its department of strategic planning and policy. One of her first assignments was to examine how legislative initiatives impact the pharmaceutical industry. To better understand the issues, Newman monitored meetings on general healthcare legislation and studied how the marketplace was changing. She also prepared presentations and recommendations for strategic operations.

Industry Nurse Checkpoint

Are you interested in broad views?

Are you a creative problem solver?

Do you like to push boundaries?

If so, read on

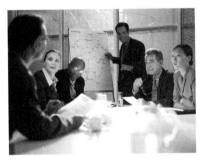

In keeping with her work as an industry nurse, Newman focused on quality improvement initiatives and worked with Human Resources on projects that involved Pfizer's employee benefits, specifically whether Pfizer should purchase healthcare collectively with other large employers. After analyzing the benefits, she recommended that Pfizer participate in a purchasing coalition. Shortly thereafter, she was asked to run the managed care program in Corporate Employee Benefits for all of Pfizer employees and their dependents in the United States. In talking about her job, Newman states that in large part she was assigned to "kick the tires" of managed care plans. Her role required assessing everything from the quality-of-care to the quality of call-answering, to the types of health improvement programs Pfizer offers employees.

In July 2000, Newman took a new position as Manager of Employer Initiatives. In Pfizer's pharmaceutical group, Newman and her team of seven are challenged with helping large employers optimize their healthcare investment. They are a dedicated group who help employers to evaluate work-site productivity, develop targeted health and wellness programs, establish screening programs to reduce absenteeism, and demonstrate the value of pharmaceuticals. All of these programs can influence the company's bottom line.

A day in the life

Newman works with on-site medical directors and employee benefits people to help develop and implement specific programs. For example, she has set up programs to screen employees for high cholesterol and diabetes. Employees who test positive for those and other conditions are provided with information on management of the condition. She is also working with the head of St Luke's-Roosevelt Hospital's Headache Program, which is located in New York City, to put in headache treatment programs at employee sites. "Migraines impact an employees' ability to work productively," she says.

On the surface, her analytical work is vastly different from general nursing, but Newman sees some connection. "Nurses work with individuals to improve their health and wellness and educate them about it. We provide a similar service to employees, plus we're working to help key decision makers with an organization to understand the disease and how to help their employees better manage it."

Profiling the job

Newman says a benefit to her line of work is that it has a positive impact on so many people. She does admit that there are drawbacks, however. "Because this is the corporate world — you are not as autonomous as you might like." She attributes this to the layers of management approval attached to getting programs off the ground, both within her own company and the companies with which she is working. Another drawback is working long hours. "No one in corporate America works nine to five," she says. "It's more like 8:00am to 8:00pm or even midnight. In corporate America you don't leave your job until you get it done. Frankly, I suspect I'd be working less hours in general nursing."

When Newman left hospital nursing, computers were just being installed on every floor. Now she spends 80 percent of her day on a computer, working up letters to potential customers, communicating with employers on current programs, and keeping abreast of current legislative and business-related developments in the media.

Newman expects corporate initiatives will increase as employers realize that good health has a positive return on their bottom line. She anticipates that Pfizer will continue to map out an agenda focused on helping employers, employees and the community at large maintain and improve their health.

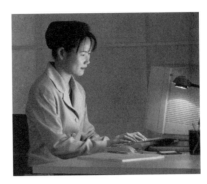

Recently Pfizer merged with Warner-Lambert to become the fastest growing pharmaceutical company in the world. In 2000, the company, whose scientific staff alone numbers around 12,000, spent an estimated $4.7 billion on research and development. Its corporate motto is: "Life is our life's work."

Newman's personal perspective on health has been shaped by her life's work. "I have a greater respect for my own health," she says. "I'm totally conscious of what I eat. I work out and make every effort to find balance in my life."

Did you know? Studies have shown that workplace programs incorporating health promotion help employees detect problems earlier, decrease absenteeism, lower turnover, increase productivity and improve morale.[1]

fast facts

What do you need?

- Ability to document activities and problem-solve
- Ability to work independently
- Effective verbal and written communication abilities

What's it take?

- A current license as a Registered Nurse (RN)
- BSN preferred, ADN usually sufficient for entry level
- A master's degree is sometimes required

Where will you practice?

- Corporate offices
- Department stores
- Shopping malls
- HMOs
- Factories
- Mills
- Health insurance companies
- Telephone triage centers

1 Bottom Line Business Health Check Up. "Trends in Health Care".
http://www.bizhealthcheck.com/trends/index.html

infection control nurse

A TRUE TALE

When Elaine Larson, PhD, FAAN, CIC, applied to college 30 years ago, nursing represented one of the great opportunities for women. It also represented a great opportunity to live out a commitment to a service profession, work with people and learn, learn, learn. Larson says her reasons for choosing nursing would be different today from what they were 30 years ago, but the career choice would be the same.

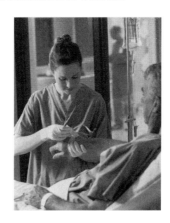

Larson, who has subsequently earned degrees in microbiology and epidemiology, entered the profession as an infection control nurse at a time when physicians were the principle practitioners and adminis-trators. Gradually, nurses assumed greater levels of responsibility for surveillance, and because of this became better equipped to care for their patients. "Today, we're more clinically in tune with what's going on at the bedside and can identify many procedures from the patients' point of view. We have a clinical appreciation to effect changes in practice and behavior," says Larson. Effecting changes in practice and behavior is the main goal of infection control nurses, who are responsible for preventing and managing the spread of infection in healthcare organizations. Before they can take proper corrective measures to limit the extent of infections and help to ensure that similar episodes are not repeated, they have to investigate the history of outbreaks and isolate sources of infection. The job has become more difficult than in the past because of the number of drug-resistant organisms, the reemergence of tuberculosis and other newer diseases, widespread travel to more parts of the globe, and the increasing number of people who are immunocompromised as a result of aging, disease and chemotherapy.

A day in the life

Unlike most nurses who care for individual patients, infection control nurses develop systems of surveillance and education activities for an entire institu-tion. They identify where problems are and how to reduce their effects and likelihood. "Sometimes it's very much like being a detective," she says. The infection control nurse also trains healthcare staffers on infection control

Infection Control Nurse Checkpoint

Do you like detective work?

Are you interested in working with data control protocols and statistics?

Would you enjoy tracking cases of infection over an extended period of time?

If so, read on

practices that range from proper hand-washing techniques to ensuring that laundry workers wear gloves when handling soiled bed linens and gowns.

"Although the infection control nurse usually reports to the executive vice president or hospital administrator for patient care services and regularly collaborates with physicians and other professionals in infectious disease, microbiology and behavioral psychology, he or she functions very much like a supervisor," says Larson. "We have free reign to correct problems." The Centers for Disease Control and Prevention (CDC) recommends one infection nurse for every 200 beds, and most hospitals adhere to these guidelines. While Larson wears a lab coat, the "uniform" of other infection control nurses depends on their hospital guidelines. While the nurses normally set their own hours within their employer's requirements, and generally on work days, if an outbreak is serious, they'll be on the scene nights and weekends as well.

Profiling the job

Most outbreaks aren't serious, but in virtually any hospital at any given time there's at least one infectious outbreak. An outbreak is defined as any occurrence above the normal rate for a specific hospital. In the children's ward, respiratory infections, viruses and chicken pox give cause for concern. In older patients, diarrhea, salmonella and infections such as MRSA (methicillin resistant staphylococcus aureus), Hepatitis B virus or mycobacterium tuberculosis are what they look out for. Cultures grown in the lab can identify potentially pathogenic organisms. Then sensitivity studies are performed to indicate antibiotics best suited to treat the organism. Some outbreaks last for several months and have multiple causes. Additionally, Larson adds, "Sixty to 70 percent of the infections that patients get in hospitals are brought in by the patients themselves. We call this their own flora."

Approximately 50 percent of an infection control nurse's day is spent examining patients and observing them for signs and symptoms of infection. These nurses also spend time on protocols, administration and education.

In her 30 years in the field, Larson has seen some unusual situations. Once she traced a staph infection to a surgeon who was unknowingly infecting his own patients. Recently,

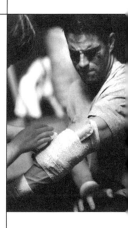

the infection control staff was able to associate nurses' artificial fingernails with harboring an organism that causes infection in premature babies. Other infection control nurses have tracked tuberculosis transferred to staff members by sick prisoners. Larson has never seen an AIDS patient infect another in the hospital but is rigid about safe handling of needle sticks and blood. "The job of an infection control nurse in collaboration with occupational health personnel is to protect the staff and patients," she says, noting that nationwide there have only been a few cases of staff acquiring HIV infection from needles carrying the disease.

Larson, who is currently the Professor of Pharmaceutical and Therapeutic Research at Columbia University School of Nursing, has worked in infection control at several hospitals around the country. Currently, she does research in the field. At Johns Hopkins University School of Nursing she directed a postdoctoral program in infection prevention and has served as a member of one of the National Institutes of Health HIV/AIDS study sections. She has also been president of the Certification Board for Infection Control, and a Fellow of the Infectious Disease Society of America. Larson chaired the CDC's Healthcare Infection Control Practices Advisory Council until summer of 2000. She has also served on the President's Committee for Gulf War Veterans Illnesses, and has been an infection control and nursing consultant in international settings such as Kuwait, Jordan, Singapore, Australia, Ghana, Peru, Brazil, Spain and Egypt. She also sits on the Clinical Research Roundtable for the Institute of Medicine.

Since Larson started in infection control nursing, the role of her specialty has greatly expanded. "We're responsible for quality assurance, risk management and practice pattern surveillance." The field that used to be focused almost entirely on hospitals now includes outpatient departments, extended care facilities, home care and clinics.

An infection control nurse can be responsible for a system of nursing homes or day care centers. In fact, about one-fifth of infection control professionals are employed at non-acute inpatient institutions, long-term care, mental health and rehabilitation facilities.

The specialty, which began in the 1960s, arose from a recommendation by the Joint Commission on Accreditation of Healthcare Organizations that

Did you know?
Nosocomial infections are a major source of morbidity and mortality, affecting more than 2 million patients annually in the U.S. The estimated annual economic cost is more than $4.5 billion.[1]

hospitals appoint infection control committees. Because of increased focus on healthcare costs, growth in the field is expected. Tracking infection rates is necessary to compare a hospital's infection experience with that of other hospitals and with itself over time, and to reduce possible infection control problems and subsequently, healthcare costs.

Larson says what she likes best about her specialty is solving problems. The worst part is the frustration of trying to convince people to change their behavior — even the simplest thing such as washing their hands, for example. "Most people know what needs to be done but it's getting them to do it that's the trick."

>>> fast facts

What do you need?
- Knowledge of state and national regulations surrounding infection control
- Experience with staff and patient inservices
- Certification in Infection Control (CIC)

What's it take?
- A current license as a Registered Nurse (RN)
- A Bachelor of Science in Nursing (BSN)
- Education at the master's level may be required

Where will you practice?
- Community or regional hospitals
- Non-acute inpatient institutions
- Long-term facilities
- Mental health facilities
- Rehabilitation facilities
- A variety of private and public healthcare, academic, or industry/consulting settings

1 Association for Professionals in Infection Control and Epidemiology (APIC).
"Infection Control — A Few Ounces of Prevention..." http://www.apic.org/html/cons/icdesc.html

long-term care nurse

A TRUE TALE

A decade ago, when Kathryn Changas, RN, was a nursing assistant in a long-term care facility, a nurse on the unit talked her into going to nursing school. "That nurse was so compassionate and caring and I wanted to be like her," the 35-year-old Changas says.

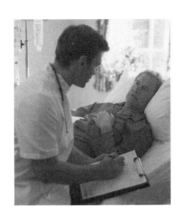

After a year she began a nursing program at Indiana University. During the four years it took to complete her BSN, she cashiered at a grocery store to pay the tuition, but through it all she never doubted she'd made the right career choice. "I had a clinical instructor in my first two years there who was very caring and had high standards which she instilled in her students. She was so proud of her profession and highly involved in it. She made nursing an art," recalls Changas.

A day in the life

Fresh out of school, Changas took a job at Bridgeview Health Care, a nursing home in Bridgeview, Illinois. For a year she was the charge nurse of its 47-bed Alzheimer's unit. Here she learned about the different activities and environmental factors that stimulated these patients and how to orient them to their environment. "I focused on spending quality time with my patients," she says.

In 1997 Changas was recruited by the Evergreen Health Care Rehabilitation facility in Evergreen Park, a suburb of Chicago. Evergreen is a 242-bed unit that specializes in wound care and rehabilitation. First she was a staff nurse, then coordinator of its 73-bed dementia unit. Soon she was promoted to assistant director of nursing, and ultimately, to director of nursing for the entire facility. In her capacity as Director of Nursing, Changas reported to the facility's administrator, and was supervisor to 75 nurses and 105 certified nurse assistants.

Residents are there voluntarily. The average stay on the short-term unit is 17 days, increasing to 45 days in the sub-acute medical complex (renal failure, wounds, amputations and post-strokes). Traditional long-term care patients suffering from strokes, seizures and COPD (chronic obstruction

Long Term Care Nurse Checkpoint

Can you be as attuned to a patient's psychosocial needs as his or her medical needs?

Would you find it gratifying to get a stroke victim back on his or her feet?

Do you enjoy being with and conversing with older persons?

If so, read on

pulmonary disorder), stay longer. 'Codes' — cardiac arrest requiring recusitation — are, unfortunately, common.

Evergreen markets itself to hospitals and social workers. It was recently bought by a company that brought in high-tech exercise equipment for the rehabilitation program. They've also made the facility more physician-driven. "Doctors are much more a part of things we do here now," says Changas.

The Alzheimer's unit is almost always full. It's $160 a day fee is covered by Medicare, Medicaid or private insurance. The youngest patient is 55. With younger adults the disease is usually more virulent and faster acting. Most patients get regular visitors but often don't recognize them, which is difficult for everyone involved. Evergreen runs both a support group and family counseling meetings to help family members better handle the situation of losing — but not losing — a loved one.

Profiling the job

Most of the activities at Evergreen are designed to create links for the patients to their earlier lives and to help them stay active where possible. For example, the activities department helped a wood worker build a birdhouse. There are exercise classes. Many residents dance without feeling self-conscious. When the television is on, it's usually tuned to old movies. There are also outings, where residents are taken to museums, to see holiday lights, and to restaurants.

Changas typically arrives at the center by 6:30am to check on the day's staffing. Problems are rare because her staffers are diligent and content. After reading the 24-hour reports, Changas and her assistant make rounds on all the units. Some rooms have one, two, three or four occupants. By 7:45am she is usually meeting with her six-person nurse management group to talk about care plans and problems. By 8:30am she meets with department heads on the facility's census, activities and incidents. She'll identify the patients in isolation due to viruses or other infections. By 9:30am she is on the floor again, making rounds and making sure that by 10:00am everyone who can

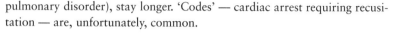

Changas says that unlike general nursing patients, those in long-term care have psychosocial needs that often outweigh their medical needs. "We offer more of an activity program than curative treatment."

Did you know? In the next 30 years, America's 65 and older population is expected to double to over 69 million. Of the 65+ population, 43 percent can expect to spend some time in a nursing home or long-term care facility.[1]

be out of his or her room is up and on the move. Next comes a meeting with her two lead CNAs, followed by a 10:00am quality assurance meeting. Team members will discuss with the dietitian nutritional plans and problems such as why residents are losing weight. Once a week she does four-hour rounds with the wound care skin doctor specialist and physical therapist. By 5:00pm, she's usually on her way home.

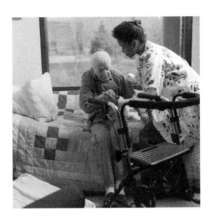

"In long-term care, we're taking them quicker and sicker from the hospitals, requiring more skilled nursing and crisis intervention."

Kathryn Changas, RN

Getting to know the patients and knowing that you're making a difference in their quality of life is what makes her job worthwhile, says Changas. She was particularly elated by a 107-year-old patient who, despite dementia, knew her and called out her name to invite her to talk whenever she passed his room.

She worries about her specialty because of the lack of interest in Alzheimer's care from most nurses. "They fear that they won't keep their skills up here," she says. "And many think it's too sad."

Changas expects that will change as more advanced practice nurses and specialty nurses get involved. They are already coming into the field, drawn by the patient mix and variety of treatments, competitive salaries and eight-hour shifts. Since she started doing this 10 years ago, she says that long-term care has become more like the medical-surgical area. Assisted living is now more like long-term care was 10 years ago. "We're taking them quicker and sicker from the hospitals, requiring more skilled nursing and crisis intervention," Changas says. Procedures like dialysis and intravenous therapy that years ago were only done in hospitals are now routinely done at facilities like Evergreen.

From her experiences, Changas has learned to better understand people's needs. The patient and his or her family are going through a grieving process and they need to talk to someone. "I'm glad to be the one they choose. Working in long-term care with the patients has made me more caring towards my own family," she says. "It's a real bonus."

PATIENT POINT OF VIEW

The hospital called to take him. He was confused and combative and they had to keep him restrained and on a mix of psychotropic drugs. Changas went to the hospital to screen him and met his wife and daughter. She listened to how the man had clumsily progressed from realizing that he had this dreadful disease, Alzheimer's, to past the point where he knew who he was. Changas, who admitted him to the facility, watched through the months as he deteriorated into only fractured moments of lucidity. He would come visit her in her office, but it was his wife who was the most grateful. With the help of the support services, she and her daughter adjusted well to "night falling" on their loved one.

>>> fast facts

What do you need?
o Medical-surgical skills with technology such as IV's, ventilators, and tube feedings
o Mentoring, teaching, and team-building skills
o Ability to view aging as a natural, dignifying process

What's it take?
o A current license as a Registered Nurse (RN)
o BSN preferred, ADN usually sufficient for entry level
o A master's degree is sometimes required

Where will you practice?
o Hospitals
o Nursing homes
o Extended care facilities
o Retirement communities
o Home-health agencies

1 HealthEssentials Inc. "Long-Term Care Industry". http://www.healthessentialsinc.com/longterm.htm

military nurse

A TRUE TALE

In 1979, when Major Matthew M. Ruest, RN, MS, was 18, he joined the U.S. Army hoping to become a paramedic. Instead, he found mentors who shaped and molded him and encouraged him to shoot higher. "They told me that the field of nursing would be more challenging and pressed me to continue my education," says Ruest. That led first to a Licensed Practical Nurse degree, then a Registered Nurse degree. It also led to one of the most satisfying careers he could ever have imagined.

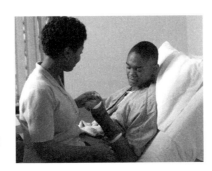

In 1980, at age 19, Ruest was posted as a senior medic in a small dispensary emergency room in Korea. One night, while he was working the late shift, a soldier in a jeep accident lost his leg. Along with the physicians, Ruest stabilized him and within the hour, had arranged to transfer him to a larger medical facility.

It was his first real experience feeling the impact one stranger can have on the life of another. Soon after, he found himself delivering babies. (Only emergency babies, of course.) He delivered the baby of a soldier's wife on the floor of their home. "At that point I'd seen one 20-minute movie on delivering," he says. "But you just do it." These experiences became opportunities for growth, and many more followed. He loved the challenging blend of responsibility and opportunity and knew he'd made the right career choice.

After Korea, Ruest returned to the U.S. His first stop was Fort Lewis in Washington, where he earned an LPN certification. A few years later, at the Eisenhower Army Medical Center at Fort Gordon in Augusta, Georgia, he staffed a surgical intensive care unit (SICU) recovery room. All the other nurses on the SICU night shift were men. This was a real eye opener for him.

A day in the life

Two years later Ruest was dispatched to the emergency room on an Army base in Augsburg, Germany. "The service was opening a new ICU facility," and at 23 years old, I was deciding what kind of equipment to put in it," he says. "It was exciting to have that kind of responsibility and to set things up the way I wanted them to be."

Military Nurse Checkpoint

Are you comfortable with the idea of periodically being isolated from loved ones?

Are you comfortable with taking orders?

Does the idea of being able to see the world in a protected, collegial atmosphere appeal to you?

If so, read on

Since then Ruest has traveled among many military hospitals, earning higher degrees, and he now has a Master in Trauma and Critical Care. "For me," he says "the Army has been an exceptional choice. I'm reminded of it daily when I realize how well I've been educated and what a real difference I can make in another person's life."

Profiling the job

Like Ruest, a good percentage of military nurses have master's degrees, especially high-ranking officers. He considers his salary competitive with a civilian's — less than he would earn in a high-risk inner-city hospital but more than in a low-risk small rural center. His benefits are incomparable, though. "In the last 20 years, the only time I ever had to worry about healthcare was the three years when I wasn't in the Army," he says. "I think our health benefits are unbeatable." And after 21 years — when Ruest is 41 — he can retire with full benefits. Then he can start a whole new career or continue as a nurse wherever he chooses. "The camaraderie that comes with working as a nurse in a military environment is different," he says. Interestingly, respect for rank doesn't cause problems. If anything, it causes people to talk to each other more. Those open lines of communications also exist between staff and patient. "Because of the common bond of being in the military, the nurse is likely to really understand the patient. But when these people become patients, we become professionals and respect both their personal and medical privacy," Ruest says. While the types of diseases a military nurse sees are similar to those in the civilian population, the patient's health and attitude differ measurably. Usually, military personnel are healthier than the general population because they're more physically fit, well-nourished, and tend to be drug free. Another plus for a military nurse is the opportunity to exercise leadership and change jobs without sacrificing seniority. The benefits are great too: education, travel, full medical, a pension after twenty years, plus a chance to serve your country.

"The Army provides the same quality of care as the outside world. In some measures, it may even be better."

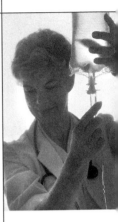

The downside is that "we're often sent away from our families on temporary duty assignments. Technically, we can negate some of these assignments, if we want to, but that may affect future career options," says Ruest. "If you want to stay in the military and get promoted you've really got to consider accepting these assignments," he says. "In the Army if you're told you have to work nights, essentially you work nights," he says. "It's a trade-off — less freedom of choice than in the outside world, but great perks and a lot of opportunity."

PATIENT POINT OF VIEW

The infantryman was crossing a street with two of his friends while on duty when an explosion nearby ripped through his body. He was brought in to surgery and then, later, to the ICU where nurses worked as a team along with the physicians to get the man's vital signs stabilized. The nurses tended to him through that first perilous night and called his family. When his parents and wife arrived at the hospital, the nurses gave them updates as to his condition and answered all of the family's questions. Weeks later, when the soldier left the hospital, he left behind a note commending his military partners for their compassion and care. "You are the true brethren," he wrote. "You make me proud to serve a country where you all are citizens."

Did you know? Over four thousand active-duty Army Nurse Corps officers provide nursing care in both inpatient and outpatient settings to approximately 524,000 active-duty service members and their beneficiaries.

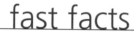

fast facts

What do you need?

- Willingness to be called for war-time duty
- Willingness to work in a highly structured environment
- Ability to work in both peace and war-time settings

What's it take?

- A current license as a Registered Nurse (RN)
- BSN preferred, ADN usually sufficient for entry level
- U.S. citizenship

Where will you practice?

- Ambulatory clinics
- Community hospitals
- Medical centers
- Hospital ships
- Field hospitals
- Military ships
- Aircraft

chapter sixteen
neonatal nurse

A TRUE TALE

At the age of 27, Debra Sansoucie, RN, EdD, CNNP, quit her secretarial job, moved to Long Island, NY and took on her dream. She began taking courses at Suffolk County Community College that would eventually culminate in an associate degree in nursing. Later, while working towards her

Neonatal Nurse Checkpoint

Can you support a parent's decision even if it's 180 degrees different from what you'd do?

Are you comfortable handling very tiny infants?

Do you like non-stop action?

If so, read on

BSN degree at the State University of New York at Stony Brook, she worked in the Neonatal Intensive Care Unit (NICU) at New York Hospital, Cornell Medical Center. Then she transferred to the NICU at Stony Brook in 1986.

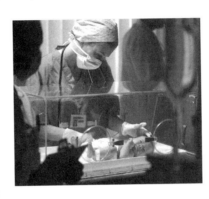

"I was always interested in newborns and intensive care. Initially, it was frightening. The 80-patient unit looked to me like a space lab station. But I was hooked right from the start." Sansoucie commuted from her home in New York to the University of Pennsylvania where she obtained her MSN degree and certification as a neonatal nurse practitioner. "As an RN I loved what I was doing but I wanted to increase my level of autonomy," she says. In 1994, while she continued to work in the NICU, Sansoucie joined the faculty of the Stony Brook School of Nursing. There she inaugurated the first Neonatal Nurse Practitioner Program in the State of New York. Sansoucie added a doctorate of education to her credentials in 1999. "Doing NICU nursing full time was too emotionally draining for me," says Sansoucie. While she felt connected with the babies and parents in her unit, she also recognized that she was having a hard time separating from them. "I doubt that I'd still be working here if I didn't have the educational aspect of my work life for reprieve."

A day in the life

Nursing sick newborns is much like acute care general nursing in medical terms, with the difference that this patient population is unusually vulnerable. "Too tiny and helpless sometimes to even exist, they truly need nursing advocacy," she says.

As a state hospital in a university town with a "United Nations-like population," Stony Brook has a large percentage of Medicaid patients.

"We see everything — including our share of babies born to HIV-positive and drug-addicted mothers. Those are the roughest." But the multiples are not easy either. She's cared for one set of quintuplets and many sets of quadruplets.

The unit is serviced by 90 nurses, nine of whom are men. The nurses and nurse practitioners generally work 12-hour shifts, but sometimes the nurse practitioners stay on duty for 24 hours straight. In addition to managing the care of the patients in the NICU, the nurse practitioners are responsible for overseeing the delivery room. They attend all high-risk deliveries, including every caesarean section. They also handle transport. If a community hospital in the region calls with a high level–needs baby, they accompany a respiratory therapist and a nurse in an ambulance to bring the baby back. "It can get very, very busy around here," laughs Sansoucie, "but I wouldn't trade it for anything."

Profiling the job

The staff nurses in the NICU usually look after two to four patients each, depending on the acuteness of the baby's condition. The unit usually has 40 or so patients, but the census has been as high as 55. For some reason,

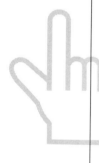

"Moms and dads are considered our patients as well as the babies themselves." Invariably, she uses her first name "to make parents feel like we're a team caring for their baby. I want them to feel that we have equal stature and want to be very reachable to them."

Christmas and summertime are exceptionally busy. Most of the patients are on high-tech equipment with monitors around the clock. The nurses feed their charges, start and maintain their IVs, draw blood, administer ventilatory care suction, and handle all manner of babies' needs. And then, too, they minister to the baby's parents.

Because of the explosion in infertility treatments and because technology has been able to save so many more babies who would have previously died of low birth weight, Sansoucie's unit has seen a major increase in the volume of patients. Multiple births that occur before the normal 40-week gestation end up there for long periods of time. "Even twins rarely go to term," she says. "Often half of our census is twins or triplets." The youngest preemie for whom Sansoucie has cared was just over 22 weeks gestation — four and a half months. "Survival at that gestation is low because the infant's lungs are not sufficiently developed to ventilate," she says. But Sansoucie was optimistic about the 25-week twins admitted to her unit that day. "Those three weeks make a huge difference," she says.

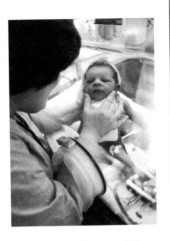

Babies born to mothers with infected placentas, toxemia, hypertension or who have had fever during labor usually go home within three to five days if there are no other complications.

Recently, after a three-month stay, the unit discharged a baby born at 27-week gestation, and weighing just over 300 grams (12 ounces). "It was the smallest one we've had here," she says. Obviously the diversity of the patient's needs and specialized care requires the nursing staff on the NICU to maintain a high level of competence in a number of challenging areas.

"Every time I see a baby who has done well, who had been very sick, I feel wonderful about my career choice," says Sansoucie. She has an opportunity every year to watch her preemies grow up at the annual picnic for the unit's graduates. "There will be a toddler there whom we thought wouldn't survive and he or she is just perfect."

One of the drawbacks of nursing seriously ill neonates is the exhausting hours. This is being exacerbated by the current shortage of nurses, leaving those in the field "caring for more and more smaller and sicker babies." There is often no salary differential for "combat pay." Another downside is the emotional drain of getting close to her patients, many of whom have negative outcomes.

Going through the grieving process with parents of a dying infant is both intensely moving and intensely maturing in the sense that "I've become more in touch with the value and joy of life," she says. "Because of my time in the neonatal unit and my experience there, I live a richer life with more gratitude and empathy than I could have imagined."

"Because of my time in the neonatal unit and my experience there, I live a richer life with more gratitude and empathy than I could have imagined."

Debra Sansoucie, RN, EdD, CNNP

PATIENT POINT OF VIEW

As a new mother, when I first saw my son in the NICU at Mount Sinai Hospital in New York City, a mass of tubes snaking around him, I thought I would break him if I touched him. This place seemed a fertile background for nightmares: If I were pregnant, I wouldn't even want to pass by. But here I was, a mother of premature twins, one of whom would die here. I watched as other parents absorbed their own version of anguish. One nurse placed a dead daughter into the arms of a father, who cradled her. Another nurse sat with a mother who was singing lullabies to her son as he wavered from this world to the next. One particularly extraordinary nurse, among a squadron of them, told me that any way you have a baby up here is a loss — through dying or the loss of the perfect birth experience. Their understanding validated that experience. Seventeen days after my "Twin A" born at 2,000 grams went home, I left humbled by the experience and grateful to the nurses who helped me through every day.

Susan Mara, Little Silver, NJ

>>> ## fast facts

What do you need?
- Supervised clinical experience in the management of newborns and their families
- Ability and desire to collaborate and consult with other health professionals in your designated specialty
- Neonatal nurse practitioners should have a master's degree in nursing with neonatal focus and often require state certification

What's it take?
- An associate's degree from a junior college (2 years) or preferably a bachelor's degree (4 years)
- A licensing exam in neonatal nursing
- There is no special program for neonatal nursing in basic RN education. Some nursing programs have an elective course and clinical rotations in neonatology

Where will you practice?
- Hospitals
- Inpatient and outpatient facilities
- Residential homes
- Family and community centers

chapter seventeen

nurse anesthetist

A TRUE TALE

Timothy Lehey, Certified Registered Nurse Anesthetist (CRNA) at the Columbia University School of Nursing in New York, has been a nurse anesthetist for 15 years. It is estimated that approximately 42 percent of nurse anesthetists are men compared to less than five percent in all of nursing. Lehey, Assistant Professor and Program Director of the Nurse Anesthesia Program, chose the specialty because of "the high level of autonomy and opportunity for better pay." While nursing salaries across the country vary widely, graduate nurses in New York City can earn an average of $40,000 a year. Graduate nurse anesthetists earn nearly double that, he says.

Lehey works in a group practice of anesthe-siologists but others in his specialty are self-employed. They work in a variety of settings from hospitals to ambulatory care centers and physicians' offices.

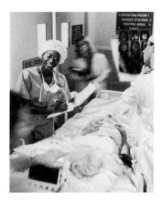

Lehey began work in 1979 as a graduate nurse. He then became a charge nurse and team leader on a 24-bed regional burn center. Later he moved on to acute care nursing in a 911-designated trauma center. He says the practice of a nurse anesthetist is very different from that of a general nurse. "First of all, we place a patient into a state of helplessness. Then we care for them, one-to-one. It's an enormous amount of responsibility when a patient's life is resting in our hands."

Do you have an affinity for pharmacology?

Do you have the stamina to work long hours?

Are you intrigued by the operating room?

If so, read on

A day in the life

A nurse anesthetist administers general, regional or local anesthesia or sedation before and during surgery or obstetrical procedures. He or she stays with the patient for the whole procedure, constantly monitoring every important body function and vital sign, changing medication to maximize the patient's safety and comfort. Nurse anesthetists analyze situations, make decisions, communicate with other members of the surgical team, and respond quickly in an emergency. Some estimate that nurse anesthetists participate in the administration of more than 65 percent of the 26 million anesthetics given to patients in the United States each year. CRNA's are licensed and can practice in all 50 states.

On a typical day Lehey arrives at the hospital around 6:30am to prepare the anesthesia machine. "I check to ensure that all parts are in order the way a pilot checks his plane before takeoff," he says. Lehey draws up the medications that will be administered during the surgery — usually eight or nine medications — and assembles the other supplies. He rarely knows when he'll leave. The type of surgery dictates the length of the operation, which could go on and on. "I've started at 7:30am, been relieved overnight and returned at 7:30am the next day to the same operation. The surgeon stayed through for 30 hours," he says. "It's not just the long hours — 12- and 24-hour shifts are not uncommon and it can be physically tiring because you're on your feet — but it's the unpredictability of it all that can wear you out. There's no assurance you'll be out at 5:00pm or 7:00pm or midnight."

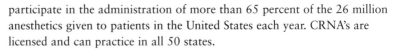

Decades ago, some physicians quipped that they could successfully perform a surgery but that the anesthesia would kill the patient. And indeed it might have. But no one is saying that today. Today, thanks to better technology, improved training of both doctors and nurses and improved pharmacology, fewer than one in 250,000 patients die in surgery as a possible or contributing consequence of anesthesia.[1]

Profiling the job

Nurse anesthetists generally pick the type of surgery that interests them, and that often determines the length of the procedure. "You can do perhaps two cardiac surgeries in a day or 10 operations in an ambulatory surgery center and be done by noon," he says. Lehey enjoys neurosurgery because it is interesting but the cases tend to be quite long.

In terms of patient stays, Lehey says, patients leave the hospital earlier than they used to. "Pharmacology has changed dramatically over the past five years. There's a tremendous push to get patients out as quickly as possible. So we give medications that provide the same analgesic relief but are shorter acting."

Nurse anesthesia requires a unique combination of technical skills and brainpower, Lehey says. "Things like how to administer a spinal or epidural anesthetic procedure, or the best place for an IV in a frail patient are very technical skills. You've got to combine that with an intellectual understanding of the ramifications of everything else you're doing."

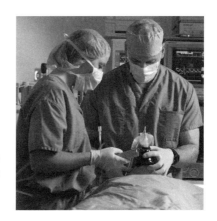

Interestingly, most lay people know little about these practitioners or what they do; they think that the practice of anesthesiology is exclusively in the hands of physicians. In fact, before World War II, it was almost entirely administered by nurses. Sister Mary Bernard, a Catholic nun who practiced in 1877 at St. Vincent's Hospital in Erie, Pennsylvania, may have been the first nurse anesthetist and St. Vincent Hospital, in Portland, Oregon, the first school of nurse anesthesia. The nurse anesthesia specialty was formally organized on June 17, 1931.

After surgery, Lehey brings the patient to the recovery room. Then, he tries to follow-up with a postoperative visit to see if the pain management was satisfactory, and to determine whether the patient can recall any aspect of the surgery or if there are any aftereffects.

While the vast majority of cases turn out well, Lehey has lost a few patients on the operating table: "They come in with three holes in their heart from a gunshot wound and there's not a lot you can do," he says. He has learned how to deal with that. In fact, he says, he's always learning new techniques, like the correct needle placement for interscalene blocks. Instead of focusing on death, he thinks about the critically ill patients approaching death who

"Things like how to administer a spinal or epidural anesthetic procedure, or the best place for an IV in a frail patient are very technical skills. You've got to combine that with an intellectual understanding of the ramifications of everything else you're doing."

Timothy Lehey, CRNA

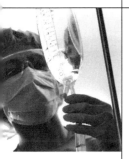

have been saved through his interventions. "It sounds very self congratulatory but the truth is that our anesthetic management does affect patient outcome." Once Lehey attended to a newborn baby whose need for a diaphragmatic hernia surgery was determined in utero. "I was awed by the potential to save this life," he says.

A bright future

There are nearly 28,000 members in the American Association of Nurse Anesthetists. Experts expect that by the year 2010, the healthcare system will need over 30,000 CRNAs. "Every week I get five to 10 flyers in the mail offering high-paying jobs," says Lehey. "All our graduates find jobs and often get to choose from four to five opportunities." Salary.com suggests that on average, salaries start around $80,000, and may top-off around $110,000, depending on the practice arrangement, geographical location and population served.

PATIENT POINT OF VIEW

Many patients worry that when they "go under" anesthesia, they may never "come out." They put their faith in the man or woman putting them to sleep. Nurse anesthetists give the drugs and, just as importantly, the moral support to help patients get through what's often a stressful situation. Their strong people skills come into play when explaining to patients the procedure as well as what can be expected afterwards.

fast facts

What do you need?
○ To graduate from a 24–36-month nurse anesthetist program (they average 28 months) that includes both classroom and clinical experience mainly comprised of:
– Courses in anatomy, physiology, pathophysiology, biochemistry, chemistry, physics and pharmacology, as related to anesthesia
– Supervised operating room experience with various anesthesia techniques and procedures for all types of surgery and obstetrics
○ At least a year of acute care nursing experience prior to entering a nurse anesthesia program
○ Those accepted often have several years of experience in intensive care nursing

What's it take?
○ A Bachelor of Science in Nursing (BSN)
○ Successful completion of a national certification exam
○ Forty hours of continuing education over a biannual period to maintain certification
○ Approximately 95% of all nurse anesthetists are certified

Where will you practice?
○ Group practice of anesthesiologists
○ Hospitals
○ Outpatient surgery centers, in collaboration with a surgeon, dentist or podiatrist
○ Self-employed

1 American Association of Nurse Anesthetists. "Quality Care in Anesthesia".
http://www.aana.com/library/qualityofcare.asp
2 "What is a Nurse Anesthetist? Introduction". http://www.anesthesia-nursing.com/wina.html

chapter eighteen
nurse-midwife

Nurse-Midwife Checkpoint

Do you see birth as a time of energy and strength?

Are you interested in providing a personalized approach to gynecological care?

Would you feel comfortable birthing in a variety of environments, including in the home, without the supplies and equipment available in a hospital?

If so, read on

A TRUE TALE

As a young girl, when Lisa Kane Low, PhD, RN, CNM, first heard about midwives, she thought they were quite medieval or gothic. Little did the now 40-year-old Detroit native know that she would become one. Low also didn't know growing up that her great-grandmother was a nurse, as was her mother before her. Despite her keen interest in issues of pregnancy and women's health during high school, Low started at Michigan State University in pre-law. Then, 20 years ago, she had a life-changing experience. "For the first time in my life I witnessed a birth firsthand. When my

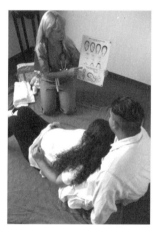

sister-in-law gave birth to my nephew, I was overwhelmed watching the midwives work," she says. "I decided then that I wanted to be one of these extraordinary people, and I have never looked back."

In 1980, Low transferred to the University of Michigan and, in 1984, she graduated with a Bachelor of Science in Nursing. After a year of working in Labor and Delivery, she proceeded directly to the University of Illinois at Chicago and left two years later with a master's degree. In 1986 she took the national boards to become a certified nurse-midwife.

"Midwives do more than just attend childbirth," says Low. "We actually function as primary healthcare providers for women, who render prenatal, intra-partum and post-partum care as well as participate in the diagnosis and treatment plans of obstetrical and gynecological problems." Some midwives, in addition to their involvement in a woman's pregnancy and childbirth, also handle annual gynecological exams, pap smears, birth control, hormone replacement and infertility problems.

A day in the life

In her 15 years of practicing nurse midwifery, Low has attended more than 1,000 births. For the last eight years she has both taught and practiced midwifery at the University of Michigan. In addition, she just completed her doctoral dissertation, which examines the adolescent's experiences of childbirth. While most people think of midwives and home birth, Low says that most women who choose midwives actually give birth in a freestanding birth center or a hospital. In fact, 96 percent of certified-midwife-attended births today are performed in hospitals. Birthing in the home, however, has been part of her experience. She says: "I've done emergency home births, but not by design," she says. "At the hospital there is much more back-up available." For example, she has access to fetal monitors, ultrasound, lab analysis, emergency equipment and auxiliary personnel as needed. But she does prefer to treat women who want "low-tech" care — fetascopes as opposed to fetal monitors, for example. She notes that between 85 to 90 percent of midwife births take place without a physician present, although one is always on call if their services are needed. Because she screens out high-risk deliveries such as insulin-dependent diabetics, emergencies are very rare.

"A midwife and obstetrician have very different perspectives on birthing," says Low. While obstetricians tend to be more technology-oriented, especially in the use of the latest equipment, midwives tend to use other time-honored, low-tech techniques — soft lights, massage, and as few high-tech accouterments as possible unless they are necessary. We do agree on one thing, however. The safety of the mother and the baby are paramount in any experience of childbirth."

Instead of using mechanical intervention — like ultrasound — to determine intrauterine growth, Low uses her own physical exam to assess the position of the fetus at each visit.

Profiling the job
As a midwife, Low employs a number of different modalities including, at times, herbs and homeopathic products, chiropractic, acupuncture and allopathic medications. She may also employ massage therapy to help manage problems. Conversation helps too. To maintain normalcy in the birthing process, Low works to develop a relationship with the family. This effect gives them a sense of safety and security, and helps her as well. She spends a lot of time with her moms-to-be during prenatal visits. Routine prenatal exams include traditional practices, such as testing urine for protein, testing

Did you know?
The cesarean section rate for hospitals with nurse-midwifery services has been about 13 percent lower than the average cesarean section rate for all hospitals.

"Midwives
do more than
attend child-
birth. They
actually
function as
family planners,
rendering
complete
prenatal, intra-
partum, and
post-partum
care."

Lisa Kane Low,
PhD, RN, CNM

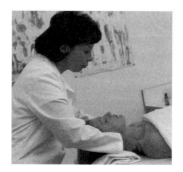

glucose, taking blood pressure, measuring the fundus and fetal heart sounds. But Low discusses nutrition and evaluates her patient's total physical and emotional well-being as well. "Whether a woman and her partner are happy about the pregnancy and how well they're getting along often influences the way a birth proceeds," she says. In essence, Low is able to combine a low-tech approach for each woman with individualized care that may use high-tech interventions, but only when truly needed. This way, a woman gets the benefit of personalized care but also has access to any of the medical procedures that could become needed for her uniquely.

Aside from midwives' renewed popularity of late, the practice has changed in that more women doubt their ability to give birth naturally and want more technology. Originally women came in to see a midwife because they wanted a drug-free birth. Now 40 to 50 percent request some sort of epidural, says Low. Part of the midwife's job is to educate women about the many options, risks and benefits that are available to them in the course of labor, so they may make informed decisions about their birth experience and their baby's well-being.

One of the challenges that often faces midwives is reimbursement. While midwife-attended births are very cost effective, many providers do not automatically cover their services. This is an issue that the profession, individually and as a whole, is increasingly looking to address.

PATIENT POINT OF VIEW

When the couple found out that she was pregnant, they were exuberant. The mother-to-be felt well and started off with her regular OB/GYN. But as the couple did more research into the birthing process, they decided to use a midwife group. They felt very comfortable with the midwife practitioner and her approach to working with them in developing a birthing plan. The couple was given plenty of time for questions and general conversation, which strengthened the relationship among them all. They both attended the prenatal course offered by the midwifery group, watched birth movies, read

"The Magical Child" and got a realistic view of the natural birthing process. When the baby didn't turn at 35 weeks, the couple worried about delivering the baby at home, but eventually he got into position and the home delivery was on. The due date came and went. Nine days later her water broke. After timing the contractions until they were five minutes apart, they paged their midwife. When the midwife arrived, she assured the expecting woman that she was making very quick progress. Finally, after many pushes, a healthy baby boy let the world know he was there with a hearty wail.

fast facts

What do you need?
- Advanced training in obstetrics and gynecology
- To pass a national certification exam
- Participation in continuing education programs

What's it take?
- A current license as a Registered Nurse (RN)
- A Bachelor of Science in Nursing (BSN)
- A master's degree in midwifery may be required in some states

Where will you practice?
- Hospitals
- Birth centers
- Private practices
- Health clinics
- Home birth services

chapter nineteen

obstetric nurse

**Obstetric Nurse
Checkpoint**

Do you have
excellent
communications
skills and
bedside
manner?

While
understanding
pathology, do
you still find
the process
of birth
extraordinary?

Can you
empathize with
post-partum
depression?

If so, read on

A TRUE TALE

As manager of the 21-bed high-risk obstetrics and gynecology (OB/GYN)
unit at Kaleida Health Corporation's Children's Hospital of Buffalo,
Barbara Neilson, RNC, faces challenges every day. Her unit handles pregnant women who have severe medical or obstetrical complications. These
complications run the gamut from tubal or ectopic pregnancies, premature
ruptured membranes, and abnormal placental placement, to diabetes and
hypertension. As a high-risk specialist, she also tends to healthy women
in premature labor who are confined to bed because the baby is too small
to deliver. Last year, in her facility 244 patients experienced a pregnancy
loss — 13 of them in full-term deliveries. When these unfortunate circumstances occur, Neilson is on hand to help
as a bereavement counselor.

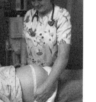

A day in the life

Her particular unit performs outpatient
gynecological surgeries as well. In some
cases procedures are done for abnormal
pap smears, and in others the work is to
help a patient with infertility. Because of
the nature of the situation, the emotional
needs of these patients and their family are
intense, particularly for the new mothers
of premature and acutely ill infants.

The average stay on the unit is approximately three to four days, but often women
can be there from a few hours (for ambulatory surgery) to several months.
The latter patients generally are those who threaten to deliver too soon,
placing the newborn at great risk. Approximately 40 percent of the long-
term patients who get labor-retarding drugs go on to full-term delivery, a
true credit to the team of 12 RNs, six LPNs and five medical assistants.

Neilson is at the nurses' station by 6:30am most mornings. First, she checks
staffing and night reports. Then she looks at the operating room schedule.
By 8:00am she is making rounds with the clinic's chief resident and
attending physicians. There are seven physicians in the group; 40 others
have practicing privileges.

At 9:00am, Neilson and her assistants begin the day's work, which will be nonstop for several hours. It includes collaborating and coordinating with other departments to arrange tests and treatments. Neilson makes rounds by herself again at 11:00am. Unlike the earlier medical rounds, this time she focuses on patient satisfaction. Is the clinic meeting the patient's and her family's needs? How is she faring emotionally? Did she really understand the earlier session with the physician? "Very often patients feel intimidated when there's a group of people at their bedsides, especially a group of physicians and nurses speaking in a foreign language — which is what our medical jargon must sound like to them. So they need help sorting it out and evaluating what was said," she says.

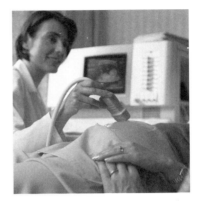

"Post-partum depression takes an extreme amount of professional caring and courtesy. As nurses, we individualize each loss with the women,"

Barbara Neilson, RNC

Later in the day, Neilson finds time for payroll review, staff scheduling, continued quality improvement projects, discharge plans, and bereavement counseling. She also attends administrative budget meetings. "Sometimes there's a little creative tension between those who allocate the money and those who want it, but there are ways to work with staff when cutbacks are needed. But it's important to be well prepared with factual numbers to defend your case," she says, "because you can be sure you'll need to."

Neilson's job doesn't end there. Woven through the day — every day — are staffing situations, like shuffling nurses from the labor and delivery floor to wherever they are needed. "In the past it was a constant challenge to make things run smoothly — but now we've got it down to a science. And when things are under control — we have more time to spend with our moms-to-be." When Neilson leaves at 4:00pm, it's often with journals and papers in hand that she didn't get to during the day.

Profiling the job

Most patients have already had initial prenatal care before coming to the high-risk unit. Although there's a mix of Medicaid and private payment patients, all patients have private rooms.

Did you know?
Nationally, as many as 30 percent of pregnancies miscarry. Although ectopics account for only a very small percent of pregnancies, Neilson says their numbers have been growing, because infertility workups sometimes result in tubal damage.

Many of Neilson's patients are under high stress — even after a successful delivery. "Post-partum depression is very real, even for healthy births. Difficult or lost births can translate into severe emotional distress," says Neilson. "They take an extreme amount of professional caring and courtesy. As nurses, we individualize each loss with the women." Neilson has strong feelings about the importance of proper care for all women and children.

"The most challenging aspects of the specialty," says Neilson, "are the financial constraints under which myself and my colleagues strive to provide high quality care. We're constantly trying to do more with less," she says. Her unit deals with it by balancing RNs with LPNs, but "there's only so much an LPN can do," she says. "LPNs can place a fetal monitor on or off but can't interpret the strip. For that a specially qualified RN is required," says Neilson. On the other hand, she adds, what is rewarding is to achieve a positive outcome — to watch a baby who has been in the unit for several weeks end up healthy and ready to go home.

Being in the high-risk unit terrified Neilson when she was pregnant with her second child. "I have seen so much and now believe that ignorance can be bliss," she says. She also believes that this is one of the times in life when all patients are vulnerable and more alike than different. "Everyone looks first to see if the baby has 10 toes and fingers and all its parts," she says. "That probably started with the birth of the very first baby."

While births have soared elsewhere in the nation, for some reason, Neilson's hospital has not experienced a baby boom. Generally, there is usually heavy volume in December. But in the year 2000, there was a crest at the end of August and start of September "nine months after the millennium," laughs Neilson.

PATIENT POINT OF VIEW
Some friends kept repeating that she was young and would have other babies, and that she should try to forget the baby girl she had just lost during delivery. Other friends, at a loss for what to say, avoided her. The only ones who seemed to know what she was going through — a crushing, breathtaking grief — were the nurses in the high-risk unit. They understood her need to grieve and although they'd seen it time and time again, were able to share the

death of dreams the young almost-mother had for this child. They knew that healing would happen slowly, but they knew too that a new pregnancy, while providing hope, would not make her forget. They realized that if she were one of the lucky ones, she'd leave this experience a more sensitive, compassionate person. They also knew that the woman wasn't alone in her grief — that her partner was suffering too — and perhaps more so in his feelings of helplessness. They listened and cared for her through this intensely distressful period.

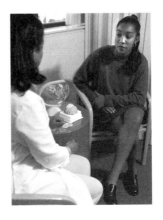

fast facts

What do you need?
- o Inpatient obstetric nurse certification may be required
- o Experience in direct patient care, education, administration, and/or research
- o CPR certification may be required

What's it take?
- o A current license as a Registered Nurse (RN)
- o BSN preferred, ADN usually sufficient for entry level
- o A master's degree may be required

Where will you practice?
- o Hospitals
- o Health departments
- o Medical offices
- o Specialty hospitals
- o HMOs
- o Clinics
- o Birthing centers
- o Nurse midwife practices
- o Home health agencies

1 Food and Drug Administration. "FDA Approves New Fetal Oxygen Saturation Monitor". http://www.fda.gov/bbs/topics/ANSWERS/ANS01014.html

chapter twenty
occupational health nurse

**Occupational
Health Nurse
Checkpoint**

Do you want
a specialty
that focuses
on wellness
and health
promotion?

Do you have a
large curiosity
to look at
someone's
health in
the context
of his job?

Are you an
effective
manager with
good judgment
and strong
nursing skills?

If so, read on

A TRUE TALE

Diane Vogelei, RN, MSN, ANP-C, became a nurse somewhat by accident. When she was figuring out what to do, the U.S. Army offered her a four-year scholarship to become a nurse. However, there was a proviso; she'd owe them three years of work after her schooling. Vogelei saw this as a double benefit though, because her training was paid for and a job was guaranteed.

Vogelei graduated in 1973 from the University of Maryland in Baltimore with a BSN, and after a stint at the Walter Reed Army Institute of Nursing, spent three years as a maternal and child health nurse in the Army, taking care of dependents and women soldiers. "I especially enjoyed the patient education and health promotion aspects," she said.

Although she enjoyed her experience in the military, Vogelei eventually moved to outpatient settings such as regular and pediatric outpatient clinics, and soon after began her family. At home, she learned how to use a computer and helped her husband, an attorney, maintain his billing program online. "I became something of a computer geek," she says. "But I felt isolated and missed nursing."

When Fireman's Fund Insurance Company was seeking a nurse with computer experience to work in its occupational health unit, Vogelei thought this could be her ideal job. After landing the position, she spent a year developing a smoking cessa-tion program, and another few years

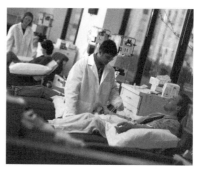

designing health-screening programs and a system to track medical leaves of absence. Vogelei was surprised by how much she enjoyed it.

In 1993, she earned an MSN from the University of California at San Francisco as an Adult Nurse Practitioner (ANP) with a specialty in occupa-tional health. When she returned to full-time nursing as an ANP, however, she realized she didn't like working evenings, nights and weekends, so she became a clinical investigator for a pharmaceutical company where the hours were more normal. Three years later, she went to work as an occupational health nurse for a company in Berkeley, CA.

In October 2000, Vogelei became manager of Employee and Occupational Health Services at the University of California, San Francisco. Her responsibilities include overall health maintenance for the facility's 6,000 health-care workers and 15,000 university employees. She reports to the unit's medical director.

A day in the life

Vogelei and her staff of four full-time nurse practitioners do about 150 health screenings a month. They review immunization status, administer flu shots, do blood pressure screenings, eye exams, spirometry tests (breathing capacity) and preplacement evaluations for certain types of employees. The most common injuries Vogelei's clinic sees include wrenched backs from construction workers, repetitive motion from clerical workers, twisted ankles and other minor injuries.

The center maintains a full-time hotline. On weekends, occupational health physicians and fellows take incoming calls. On one occasion, a call came from a staffer who had been pricked by a needle from a patient with HIV. "Based on scientific research that's available, a certain medicine can abort possible infection if given within one hour of exposure, so even in a workplace setting emergency care is important," she says.

Profiling the job

An occupational health nurse acts as "gate-opener" for health services. At work sites, this can include emergency medicine, preparation of accident reports, and coordinating further care, if necessary. They also offer health counseling, assist with health examinations and inoculations, and assess work environments to identify potential health or safety problems. Whether it's setting noise controls to prevent hearing loss, coping with stress and burnout in the workplace, or working on risk reduction of field workers, the occupational nurse is on the job.

Removing sutures, changing a burn dressing, conducting annual vision tests, assessing ergonomic issues, following up on a workers' compensation claim, and meeting with rehabilitation specialists to get an employee back on the job sooner are all component parts of occupational health nursing.

Vogelei's unit participates in research studies. One in particular was designed to develop post-exposure prophylaxis treatment options for patients with the HIV virus. Another was designed to look at clinical assessment tools used to diagnose carpal tunnel syndrome, a common workplace ailment.

The University's health services unit operates at a different pace than regular outpatient clinics, which generally require nurses to see a patient every 15-20 minutes, says Vogelei. "We often can spend up to 45 minutes per new injury and 30 minutes for routine follow-ups. A lot of the time is spent on educating the patient. For a back injury, for example, we often teach them how to care for themselves to avoid re-injury. For repetitive motion problems, we investigate proper ergonomics and urge workers to take a break every 20 minutes. We also teach them relaxation exercises."

Her hours are 7:30am to 4:00pm, Monday through Friday, for which she "probably makes 30 percent more money" than she would elsewhere. "You're not going to get rich here, but at least you have a life," she says.

It is not a life entirely shielded from empathic pain and loss, however. Her clinic is often the first stop for serious illnesses that are referred to specialists. The best thing about being an occupational nurse, Vogelei says, "is the normal life you can live because of the hours." Another plus is its emphasis on patient education and health promotion — not just treatment of injuries. "By looking forward, we can really make an impact on someone's life," she says. Being on staff also means having the power to take action. "In a regular setting, a nurse can really just counsel. But here we can do an ergonomic evaluation and then get the proper equipment to benefit the life of everyone in a department."

The worst thing, she says, is the legal aspect. "We deal with a lot with worker's compensation." That means that when she wants to order a test or send a patient to a specialist, she and the patient must wait for approval before they can do anything. "Unless we refer them to an outside healthcare provider, our hands are tied and that's very frustrating," she says.

"In a regular setting, a nurse can really just counsel. But here we can do an ergonomic evaluation and then get the proper equipment to benefit the life of everyone in a department."

Diane Vogelei, RN, MSN, ANP-C

An occupational health nurse's job changes with societal needs. Technology has meant a sharp increase in the number of repetitive motion injuries. Violence spilling into the workplace has mandated more prevention and counseling programs. Increasing diversity means possible language barriers and cultural differences. Vogelei expects occupational health services to expand to cover workers without outside insurance coverage and part-timers, despite employers' attempts to contain costs.

PATIENT POINT OF VIEW

Six years ago a campus worker got stuck with a needle and contracted HIV. Vogelei had to break the news to him and spent a good deal of time explaining the progression of the disease and preventative methods to help keep it at bay. She pulled together a group of supporters to help him in all areas of his life and set up a visitor system for him. For years after he left the center, she remained in touch with him. Once he told her, "I'm not glad this happened, but I'm glad you were there when it did." Vogelei says she has lost a lot of sleep over that experience but is glad that she was there for him.

Did you know? Sixty-five percent of Occupational Health nurses work alone.

fast facts

What do you need?
- ○ 4,000 hours of practice
- ○ Fifty contact hours in continuing education per year
- ○ Post-graduate education may sometimes be required

What's it take?
- ○ A current license as a Registered Nurse (RN)
- ○ BSN preferred, ADN usually sufficient for entry level
- ○ COHN (Certified Occupational Health Nurse) certification

Where will you practice?
- ○ Factories
- ○ Mills
- ○ Corporate offices
- ○ Department stores
- ○ Shopping malls
- ○ Hospitals

chapter twenty-one
oncology nurse

Oncology Nurse Checkpoint

Do you believe that a diagnosis of cancer is not a death sentence?

Are you at peace with the concept of death?

Can you take care of your own emotional and physical well being in the face of great sadness?

If so, read on

A TRUE TALE

"An oncology nurse never knows what the end result will be for his or her patients," says Agatha Wilkos, RN. "When my patients go through chemotherapy and return for follow-ups, I'm always wondering: 'Has the cancer come back?'" Wilkos says that people constantly ask her how she can work in an arena where sadness abounds. While admitting that many cancer patients do die, she says that this is an area where good nurses can make a difference and that there are many more positive outcomes. "Today, a diagnosis of cancer is not a death sentence."

She likes being able to establish long-term relationships with patients; with surgical nurses, it's often a mentality of prepare for the operation, heal and put it behind you. "Our patients undergo treatment for six months or longer, so I get to see them over time. You become invested in them," she says. "You watch them battling this disease and you want it to work out for them. To me, it's like a sporting event where you're furiously rooting for the outcome." In the beginning when "your team" loses, it's hard, Wilkos admits. "But in time, you know and accept that death is what happens where there's life. We're all going to die, and sometimes my goal is to help them through treatment and make their experience as comfortable as possible."

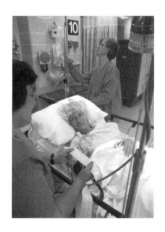

A day in the life

Wilkos earned a BSN from the University of Connecticut in 1997. After two-and-a-half years nursing in the oncology unit at Yale, the 25-year-old decided to see the United States. Her first 13-week stop was at St. Anthony's Hospital in Littleton, Colorado.

On a typical day on the medical-oncology floor, Wilkos tends to five patients. (On the night shift she'll look after up to a dozen.) One patient has just come in for the first course of chemotherapy. Wilkos explains the procedure, places the IV, draws blood, and teaches the patient about possible side effects of the medicine. Another patient is grappling with an infection, which is a common side effect of chemotherapy, because treatments compromise the patient's immunologic systems. A third patient, suffering from colon cancer, has developed a bowel obstruction that needs intervention.

Profiling the job

Wilkos estimates that approximately one-fourth of the cancers she treats originate in the breast with another quarter emerging from the prostate. Five percent of patients suffer from hematological malignancies such as leukemia, and 30 percent from lung cancer. The rest are a collection of cancers of the tongue, mouth, throat, stomach, pancreas and colon.

Every patient is different in the way he or she wants to be treated, says Wilkos. "Some want to be bombarded with information and come in with material they've downloaded from the Internet. Often, they'll know more than you do," she says. "Others just want to be hooked up, get their medication and not know what's going on. This type of patient though, is increasingly rare as more and more oncology patients want to know and be involved in their treatment."

And more and more, treatment is evolving. "Outcomes are radically different now than they were even a few short years ago," she says. New cancer drugs and protocols for treatment are constantly being introduced, often with better efficacy and side effect profiles than older ones. The majority of patients are being treated as outpatients. They get their treatments and leave, and some patients are even getting chemotherapy at home after visiting nurses set up an infusion pump. One patient has been on a 30-day drip, but it's on her own turf, says Wilkos. "I don't know if in my lifetime that all cancer will be beaten, but I do believe that eventually that day will come. We still have a long way to go, but we've come such a long way."

"In this discipline, most of our patients experience problems from both the treatment and the disease. Approximately 60 percent get chemotherapy, which can generally be administered as an outpatient procedure. However, some regimens require continuous therapy for 96 hours," says Wilkos.

"I don't know if in my lifetime that all types of cancer will be beaten, but I do believe that eventually that day will come. We still have a long way to go but we've come such a long way."

Agatha Wilkos, RN

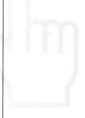

Wilkos says she feels herself hardening to the pain she sees daily. She is getting used to it, but a lot of it "still gets to" her. Often on her half-hour drive home she cries. But that time frame is "enough to help me put those feelings elsewhere," she says.

Wilkos still keeps in touch with one patient — an attorney in his 60s — who three years ago had a sarcoma in his leg. They became friends in the hospital and remained so when he went into remission. They write to each other frequently, phone and lunch together at least twice a year.

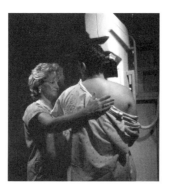

But on the other hand, she is haunted by the memory of a shy 21-year-old man with leukemia. "I was 23 at the time and he could have been anyone I knew," she says. He had so many plans. Wilkos was his primary nurse, assigned to him each time he was admitted. In June, a colleague told him not to worry and that they'd get him back on the ski slopes that winter. Soon after, he went to California for an experimental treatment and Wilkos often wondered what happened to him. Then one day she opened the local paper and there was his obituary. "He never did get back to the slopes," she says quietly. His death and that of many of her patients, has made Wilkos not as afraid of death as she used to be. "Seeing people die has given this uncertainty closure. I do feel spirits go on."

It's also made her more appreciative of the hand she's been dealt. "Sometimes I really have to ask myself if the little things I complain about are really worth the angst. I think to myself, 'I'm sure the patient in that bed would love to change places with me and complain about locking the keys in the car again.'"

PATIENT POINT OF VIEW

As a cancer survivor I am deeply indebted to many people who, in a host of important ways, assisted my recovery. One of those whose presence was a treasure was my oncology nurse, Agatha Wilkos, RN, who, by skill and training, provided expert medical treatment. But, by holding my hand in comfort when I was nearly overwhelmed by the depressive effects of chemotherapy and radiation, gave much more than that required in nursing school. For such care, I will be forever grateful.

Attorney Dale P. Faulkner, Shewville, CT

fast facts

What do you need?
- Ability to cope with human suffering, emergencies, and other stresses
- Knowledge of the nature and treatment of oncological diseases
- Knowledge of bereavement counseling techniques

What's it take?
- A current license as a Registered Nurse (RN)
- BSN preferred, ADN usually sufficient for entry level
- O.C.N. certification

Where will you practice?
- Specialty hospitals
- Medical offices
- Ambulatory care centers
- Patient homes

chapter twenty-two
palliative care/hospice nurse

**Palliative Care/
Hospice Nurse
Checkpoint**

Do you have a
strong spiritual
concept and
sense of self?

Do you have
good balance
in your own
life, so as
not to be
pulled under
by sadness?

Is it as
important to
give someone
a "healthy"
death as it is to
"cure" them?

If so, read on

A TRUE TALE

When Nancy English, PhD, APN, CS, was seven years old, her doll broke and she bandaged its head. That year her mother sent out the family Christmas card with a picture of Nancy wearing a nurse's cap, tending to the doll. Growing up in Tennessee, that image stayed in her memory. "After that, what else could I do but become a nurse?" English says.

After her first year in college, English entered into a nursing school in California. Here she earned a BSN, master's and PhD, "amassing letters after my name to deflect insecurity," she laughs. English gravitated towards

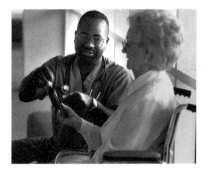

palliative care despite the fact that people don't know what it is, she says. The word palliative is derived from Latin, meaning to 'cover' or 'cloak.' In people who have been diagnosed with a life-threatening illness, the practice involves mitigating symptoms of pain and anxiety rather than addressing their cause.

A day in the life

Hospice is a method of treatment to provide palliative care for patients who are terminally ill. Dr. English is striving to "move hospice upstream to the point of diagnosis" for all individuals with a life-threatening problem. Palliative care incorporates the mind, body and spirit and includes the family in the care plan. In English's world, nurses are "partners" with physicians, patients, patients' families and other professionals, including social workers, pharmacists, chaplains and nursing assistants. The organization of this interdisciplinary team is circular, with the nurse expert acting as coordinator.

English earned a BSN with an emphasis in Public Health Nursing from the University of Southern California. Four years later, she earned an MSN as an advanced practice nurse. She received her Ph.D. in counseling psychology from the University of Humanistic Studies and later became a clinical nurse specialist in gerontology.

It was her caregiving experience with her mother and later with a 91-year-old man that highlighted the importance of palliative care. "I felt like I was being held together by a group of angels when my mother entered the hospice service shortly before she died. The nurses recognized my stress from caring for our family as well as for my mother, in addition to working full-time. I knew then that this was the field for me."

Profiling the job

English exercised her dedication and autonomy on a recent day when she drove 40 miles to visit a 67-year-old man with acute leukemia and extensive bleeding from his bladder. He was in intense pain, unable to pass blood clots through his catheter. After English taught his family how to irrigate the catheter, she urged his family to reminisce with him about the good things in his early life. "I helped manage the patient's pain and empowered the family to get on with life," she says. English feels that only a quarter of patients with a "mortal illness" acknowledge that their end is near. Most think they'll rebound after a short time.

English likes to practice direct patient family care, and also spends a good part of her professional time teaching, overseeing grants and writing about palliative care. For example, she has been working with the University of Colorado, which recently received a grant from the National Cancer Institute for a palliative care nursing education model for nurses in Colorado.

English says that in the palliative care world, nurses are "partners with physicians, with patients and their families and with other professionals such as the pharmacist, social worker and nurse's aid. It's more a circular structure than a hierarchy, with nurses at the center."

English's patient visits are paid for by the Hospice of Metro Denver through the Medicare Hospice benefit. Justifying a patient's care to fiscal intermediaries like Medicare, Medicaid and HMOs is challenging to her. "There's loads of paperwork documenting what you do, but it's worth it in the end. It's the only way to get reimbursed," she says.

English has witnessed the passing of many patients — and has her own fix on them. "What others call delirium, I call 'death bed visions,'" she says. Often as someone is ready to die, they may talk to unseen relatives who have already passed on. The patient may suddenly announce "they're here," or tell her they are being called home or that those on the other side are

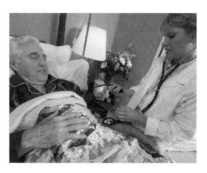

"opening the door." This often goes on for hours. "I explain what these visions are and reassure the patient and family not to be afraid," she says. "I try to make them comfortable with their loved one."

Despite the obvious ache, English feels there are many episodes that reinforce her commitment to palliative care. For example, three years ago, she admitted to the hospice a Hungarian refugee dying of colon cancer, whose ex-wife had moved back in with him to help him cope. They told her about the hardships he had endured at the hands of what they thought a confusing medical system; she patiently suggested ways to solve each problem. "Where have you been?" the woman sighed in gratitude. After English intervened, the patient lived for three more months with minimal pain or nausea, enjoying some quality time with his family.

The hospice movement started in the mid-1970s, with the first hospice established at Yale University. But it wasn't until the 1990s that the broader palliative care movement began. Currently, there are around 100 palliative care nursing specialists with advanced degrees in the United States. English anticipates there will be many more, but notes that politics greatly affect it. "There's a move to change the structure to include more palliative interventions under Medicare guidelines," she says, noting that now a lot is reimbursed through private fundraising. Medicare reimburses 80 percent of hospice stays. Although English expects that in the next 20 years palliative care will be covered through a variety of funding agencies, the national average stay in hospice is 21 days.

Surrounding herself with people with life-threatening diseases has made English calm about her own mortality. "Now, I view death as something to look at, like birth, a sacred moment when time stands still. To me, it's mystical and amazing."

"Palliative care encompasses true healing by searching for the dynamics. You don't just medicate and leave."

Nancy English, PhD, APN, CS

Profiling the job: Hospice Nurse

Sue Ann Montfort, RN, CHPN, got into hospice nursing almost by accident. "I thought it would be too depressing," she says, "but I tried it and found it overwhelmingly rewarding." That was 21 years ago. With her RN from Broward Community College and certification as a hospice nurse, she now serves as a staff nurse in the Admissions Department for Hospice By The Sea in Boca Raton, Florida. In the course of her duties over two decades, she has personally supported more than 1,000 patients through their dying process, which she says has been "a truly profound experience."

Montfort, whose own mother and mother-in-law died in hospice care, says she has learned how to honor the way each of her patients chooses to go through the process. She has also found that most people do not fear death itself as much as they fear what they may have to experience along the way. For this reason, controlling a patient's pain is one of the top priorities for a hospice nurse, and Montfort has seen many advances over the years. Now, as the disease or condition progresses and takes its course, pain medication can be adjusted accordingly, with the result that as patients get 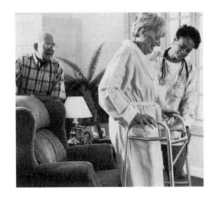 weaker, they sleep longer, and ultimately die in their sleep. "It's not the way it is in the movies," she says. "There's no reason why a patient has to endure pain."

While hospice care may take place within a hospice facility itself, 90 percent of hospice patients are cared for in their homes or other residential facilities by a team of hospice professionals. This team includes the patient's physician, the hospice nurse, a social worker, and spiritual counselor, all designed to provide patients and their families the physical, emotional, and spiritual support so beneficial for compassionate end-of-life care.

To be admitted into a hospice program in accordance with Medicare guidelines, life expectancy must be diagnosed as six months or less. Cancer patients can be ambulatory; dementia patients must be unable to eat or converse. Montfort visits four to five patients a day, and finds that one of the most troubling trends in recent years is how late in the process doctors are referring their patients into a hospice program. "Even though we can provide patients and their families a great deal of comfort in the final days, over and over I hear families say after their loved one has died, that they regret not being in the hospice program weeks, even months, earlier for the physical, emotional and spiritual relief they could have had much sooner," she says.

As for the working relationship with physicians, Montfort says the hospice nurse is "often the eyes and ears for the doctor, especially when a patient is homebound." In this way, nurses and physicians work cooperatively to manage complex situations. "It is the resolution that makes my work so worthwhile," Montfort concluded. "You go to their home, see a patient who is in pain and you get the pain under control. Next you work on the emotional aspects." She recently helped a man estranged from his family reconcile and reunite with them before he died. "The person you see die is not the person you saw when you walked in. There is no reward like it in the world."

PATIENT POINT OF VIEW

The old woman's breathing had slowed, her color changed and she wouldn't eat. She seemed agitated. The hospice nurse had invited her children to spend all the time they wanted at her bedside. When they left, the nurse returned to hold the dying woman's hand, to sing to her a song she'd heard the woman's daughter sing. The woman listened. Even her struggle to breathe relaxed as the nurse sang. As the notes softly trilled, the son and daughter returned and saw a look of peace cross their mother's face. The nurse then slipped the son's hand into the mother's to replace her own. This hospice nurse had not just cared for their beloved mother, but made them part of her care as well.

fast facts

<<<

What do you need?

- Hospice & Palliative Nurses Association (HPNA) offers certification after at least two years of experience in hospice and palliative nursing and an exam
- 710 hours of clinical practice in order to gain a palliative care nurse practitioner certification
- Expertise in pain management, issues of loss and grief, ethical and legal issues surrounding end-of-life care

What's it take?

- A current license as a Registered Nurse (RN)
- BSN preferred, ADN usually sufficient for entry level
- A master's degree in nursing

Where will you practice?

- Hospitals
- Nursing homes
- Hospices
- Private homes
- Inpatient and outpatient settings

chapter twenty-three

pediatric nurse

**Pediatric Nurse
Checkpoint**

Do you like
the energy
of children?

Are you
interested in
"getting on
their level"?

Do you see the
patient as the
family as well
as the person
in the bed?

If so, read on

A TRUE TALE

When Mary Olszewski, RN, was in high school in Philadelphia, a friend's sister who was a nurse chauffeured her back and forth to school. Her work-related stories fueled Olszweski's imagination. As a result, she volunteered at Children's Hospital and continued to work with children through college at the University of Scranton. There, she received a BSN in 1994.

For the next two-and-a-half years she worked on the medical-surgical unit at New York University Medical Center. Three-and-a-half years ago, still at the same hospital, the 28-year-old Olszewski transferred to pediatrics. In pediatrics, she says, "it's not just the one in the hospital who's the patient, it's the whole family. As a nurse, you're in the midst of everyone — but I focus mostly on the children, no matter how ill they are. Children are so vibrant and open to anything. Their energy rubs off on you."

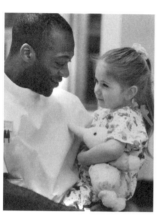

A day in the life

Currently, Olszewski is working with oncology patients while studying to be a pediatric nurse practitioner. When she finishes, she'll have prescriptive abilities and more autonomy with patients. She will then do primary care setting diagnosis and treatment, primarily of children, "evaluating and guiding families so they understand what to expect as far as growth and development are concerned." In the hospital, she sees them through specific episodes. Her 34-bed unit is filled almost all the time with both temporary residents and outpatients.

For each shift there are five or six day nurses and at night, four or five. Many children are admitted in the morning and have a range of surgeries and procedures. These include cleft lip repair, cardiac tests, tonsillectomy, or bowel and bladder surgery. The children with cancer are usually admitted if they are to have chemotherapy. "Very few children die in a hospital," says Olszewski. When palliative care becomes the option chosen by the family, children are discharged to receive hospice care at home. With this option, they are able to receive the medical care they need and still can be surrounded by loved ones in a more personal setting.

But whether the diagnosis is life threatening or simple surgery, Olszewski enjoys empowering the family by teaching coping skills for after a child's discharge. "It's gratifying to move a patient and her family a step closer," she says. "It makes me feel like I've accomplished something when I leave work at the end of the day." Olszewski involves the child, whenever possible, in his or her own care. "With some procedures, there are no choices, in which case you explain to the child as

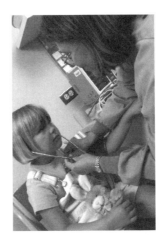

much as you feel necessary. I always tell them that any procedures are done for their benefit." Olszewski always uses her first name with her patients and lets them get to know her. "I want them to be comfortable as I examine them — and learn that in me they have a friend."

Profiling the job

In the short time she has been in pediatrics, Olszewski has seen much more routine pediatric care handled outside the hospital. Those who are admitted to the hospital are generally sicker children. "Today, children are only admitted to the hospital if it's absolutely necessary," she says. "Early puberty and sexuality, increased drug use, eating disorders and violence among younger children will impact pediatric primary care," she adds.

But these issues will have more of an effect on her when she is in the primary care setting functioning as a pediatric nurse practitioner. Now she's immersed in helping oncology families throughout their treatment. Olszewski considers this experience a wonderful opportunity. "Things I thought were terrible, I now see differently. I've gained a new perspective," Olszewski says. She also has resolution. "I take away something different from each family I work with and use it to help my next family."

"I allow the child to make choices when possible. But with some procedures, there are no choices available. Here, you need to explain to the children that these things are done not to punish them, but for their benefit."

Mary
Olszewski, RN

PATIENT POINT OF VIEW

She had been in the same hospital several times in the last two years, far from her home and parents. Because of the distance and the other children at home, her parents didn't come to visit her that much and the 11-year-old often felt desolate. Several of the nurses tried to get close to her, but one in particular became a very good friend to her. This nurse always made sure that the girl was on her roster when she was working and no matter how busy she was, she'd find time to sit on her bed and talk. Sometimes she would stay with the girl at night when she was having a bad time. The last time she left the hospital the young girl wrote to "her best friend" to let her know that she loves her like her own mom and that one day she would be a friend like that to someone who needed her.

>> > fast facts

What do you need?
- Ability to function independently
- An affinity for children
- Ability to handle lack of patient cooperation

What's it take?
- A current license as a Registered Nurse (RN)
- BSN preferred, ADN usually sufficient for entry level
- CPN (Certified Pediatric Nurse) certification may be required

Where will you practice?
- Hospitals
- Clinics
- Long-term care facilities
- Community
- Home care agencies

chapter twenty-four

pediatric palliative care nurse

A TRUE TALE

As the oldest of five children of an electrical contractor and homemaker, pediatric palliative care nurse Susan M. Huff, RN, BSN, never imagined that when she grew up she'd be cradling dying children and comforting their parents.

In the late 1970s, after two years of studying physical therapy in college, she decided she wanted to work in a different area of the medical profession. She was seeking flexibility in scheduling and a good salary. In 1982, she graduated from D'Youville College in Buffalo, New York, with a degree in nursing. There was an opening at Roswell Park Cancer Institute in the Pediatric Unit working afternoons and she decided to take it, despite her initial anxiety.

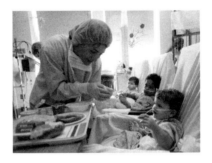

Eighteen years later, she has been an important presence to well over one hundred children, infants and adolescents at the times of their death. "The way in which you and your colleagues work together with children and their families to become one family is so gratifying," Huff says. "Even in the worst possible situation, where a parent outlives a child, there is a way to extract something positive."

A day in the life

Since 1997, Huff has headed one of the country's leading children's palliative care programs, Essential Care in Cheektowaga, New York. The program, which was founded in conjunction with Children's Hospital of Buffalo and Roswell Park Cancer Institute, has the backing of the Health Care Financing Administration (HCFA). HCFA recognized Essential Care as one of five model pediatric programs in the country, and awarded $280,000 in federal grant money to the New York State Department of Health and Essential Care. This money will be used to evaluate the effectiveness of Essential Care and to develop additional pediatric palliative care programs across New York State.

The Essential Care Team includes four staff nurses, two social workers, a child life specialist (who cares for the emotional needs of the sick child and siblings), pastoral care and bereavement specialists. They treat 30 to 40

Pediatric Palliative Care Nurse Checkpoint

Do you believe that offering comfort is as critical as offering a cure?

Are you interested in working with a team to address medical, emotional, psychological, and spiritual needs?

Do you believe the unit of care includes the entire family and not just the patient?

If so, read on

"I consider it a privilege to be allowed into these families' lives, to experience the relationship between them and their dying children. It has taught me that every second is precious and that there is joy in any given circumstance."

In 1982, while working on the pediatric unit in Roswell, she faced more primitive circumstances than she does now. Often she had to transport medical equipment in the trunk of her car and pound nails into walls or mantels to hang IV drip bags. Now she has allies — therapists and social workers who join her on visits to the children's homes where equipment has already been sent. "We're all equal partners, working as members of a supportive interdisciplinary team," says Huff.

patients a month and are often there from the time the diagnosis is made. The program's social worker has provided counseling for many families and assisted with contacting foundations for financial aid, arranging for hospital parking passes, reimbursement from the American Cancer Society for gas mileage to the hospital, and getting wheelchairs repaired.

The best thing about the specialty, Huff says, is "enlightenment." She is often asked by parents what it is going to be like at the end — what they can expect, and what they should do.

Profiling the job

Huff, who is 40, is always on call; sometimes she drives more that a 100 miles a day. A full day as a home care nurse usually entails four different home visits a day, each lasting about an hour. Afterwards, she meets with other team members from different disciplines to develop care plans. Most patients remain in her care and with the same health-care team until the end, or until the child gets better.

Indeed, not all the children she sees are dying. One in five survive their illness, and no longer need the home care Huff provides. "They have beaten the odds," she says with evident satisfaction. But those are not always the

Did you know? It is estimated that each year in the U.S., 55,000 children die from accidents, prematurity, illness or hereditary disorders.

patients who have won a permanent perch in her consciousness. There are four children who remain near and dear to Huff and she corresponds with their families every year on the anniversary of the child's death.

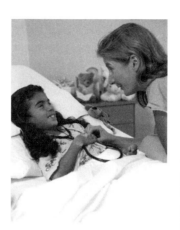

"Not having lived it, theirs is a grief I cannot understand," says Huff, whose children are ages eight and 14. "However, I do know that although the grief never goes away, at a certain point, it changes."

Experiencing a child's death is actually not the worst aspect of her job, Huff says. Rather, it's when she and the physician first tell the parents that there is a possibility that the child won't survive the illness. "It is no easier now to say those words than it was when I began."

Things have changed since Sue Huff started in pediatrics. "Our types of patients have expanded from children who have cancer to include infants born with anomalies, neuro-degenerative diseases, trisylia-13, birth asphyxia, and left heart syndrome. And the needs of the families are far more intense, because so many of the children live in divorced or foster homes."

Huff expects that in the near future, medicine will increasingly recognize the benefit of palliation and intervention. "We will do our part so that the children will be able to get on with their lives," Huff says.

PATIENT POINT OF VIEW

One mother was unsure whether to keep her young son at home to die, or bring him to the hospital. Huff sat with the mother, held her and let her talk. When she could tell from the way the little boy was breathing that it was near the end, she adjusted his medicine, dimmed the lights, and gathered the family around. She placed the child in his mother's arms. "Look how emaciated he is; look at what the cancer has done," his anguished mother said. Huff asked the boy's mother to close her eyes. "Here's what I see when

Did you know?
Just two decades ago, pediatric hospices were a rarity in the U.S. In 1983, only four of 1,400 hospices accepted children. Today, of the 2,500 hospices nationwide, 247 have programs that serve dying children.

I come into your home," Huff said. "It isn't a boy I see whose body is ridden with cancer, but a beautiful young man so loved, whose mother gave him the gift of dying at home in his own bed in his mother's arms." Later, after the boy had died, the mother told Huff that what got her through it was looking in the boy's eyes and seeing the reflection of her own love.

>>> # fast facts

What do you need?
- Hospice & Palliative Nurses Association (HPNA) offers certification after at least two years of clinical experience and an exam
- Expertise in pain management, issues of loss and grief, and ethical and legal issues surrounding end-of-life care
- CPN (Certified Pediatric Nurse) certification

What's it take?
- A current license as a Registered Nurse (RN)
- BSN preferred, ADN usually sufficient for entry level
- A master's degree in nursing

Where will you practice?
- Hospitals
- Hospices
- Private homes
- Inpatient/outpatient settings

chapter twenty-five
perioperative
(operating room) nurse

A TRUE TALE

When Patricia Seifert, RN, MSN, CRNFA, FAAN, was 25 years old, she had a death in her family that affected her profoundly. Seifert had earned a BA studying history at Trinity College, in Washington, DC, and was working as an administrative assistant, helping to support her child and husband in graduate school. The family crisis shook her up emotionally and directionally. "It made me think about life and what you do with it. I resolved then and there that I wanted to do some good, something for society," she says.

Seifert, who lived for a while in Italy but spent most of her childhood in New Jersey, decided on nursing. "If I needed it, I would always have a job

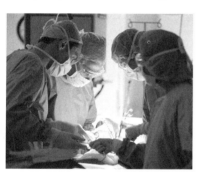

to support my children," she thought. Seifert attended Northern Virginia Community College in Annandale, Virginia. When she emerged with an ADN degree she knew she wanted to work in the operating room (OR).

In 1976, just out of nursing school, Seifert responded to an advertisement that offered to train perioperative nurses at Fairfax Hospital in Falls Church, Virginia. After a six-month course, she was put in charge of the Otorhinolaryngology Unit, the area that handles ear, nose and throat surgeries. A year later, she became head nurse for cardiac surgery there, and spent 10 of her 24 years thereafter as a cardiac operating room nurse.

A day in the Life

On a typical day, Seifert arrives at the hospital by 6:00am. She makes sure the needed equipment is functioning properly and reviews the planned procedure and her role in surgery. She goes over the lab work, blood ordered and patient consent forms. In the pre-induction area, after putting on scrubs, she may start an IV, meet and greet patients, and answer any final questions they may have before surgery.

"In the OR, you need to make immediate decisions," says Seifert. "The status of patients changes quickly. You need someone with great skilled confidence

Operating Room Nurse Checkpoint

Are you comfortable making immediate decisions?

Do you like the world of the operating theater?

Would you enjoy working closely with surgeons, anesthesiologists, and technologists?

If so, read on

to make fast decisions and deliver fast, accurate assessments." More often than not, surgical team members have Type A personalities. But because they work together constantly and interact for long periods of time, they tend to have well-orchestrated partnerships. This works well for all and on behalf of the patient on the OR table.

Almost all patients come into the OR awake, though they have been given a sedative earlier. Seifert positions the patient on the operating table, washes the surgical site in preparation for the operation, and drapes the patient with a sterile covering.

Profiling the job

Seifert's day is varied. During an eight-hour shift she can attend as few as two coronary bypass operations or as many as five hernia repairs. In addition, Seifert may participate in breast biopsies, orthopedic surgeries and gynecological procedures.

Operating room nurses are usually assigned to one room, predicated on the kinds of patients who will be in that room and the nurse's expertise. Some days he or she may work with the same surgeon throughout, and on other days there might be a different surgeon for each procedure. Seifert gets the next day's schedule the day before, but schedule changes are common. "You need to be comfortable with change," she says. And change is what she does often, rotating from scrub nurse on some procedures, to RN First Assistant (RNFA) helping the surgeon, or to circulating nurse. A scrub nurse or first assistant works directly with the surgeon within the sterile field, passing him or her sponges and other instruments during the course of the operation. An RNFA assists the surgeon by performing such tasks as controlling bleeding, providing wound exposure, and suturing during the actual procedure.

Seifert considers how strongly they shake her hand, the tonal color of their skin — which tells their oxygenation. She inquires when they last ate (to protect from aspiration) and if they have any allergies.

The circulating nurse brings the outside world to those in the sterile field, says Seifert. When she works as a circulating nurse, she watches the anesthesia monitors and ventilator settings, adjusts equipment, orders blood, x-rays or lab work and responds to any callers beeping the surgeon. She also alerts the post-anesthesia care unit or intensive care unit to prepare them for the patient's arrival, and to advise them if there are special drugs required or other needs.

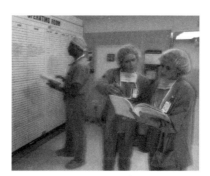

After surgery, Seifert takes the patient to the recovery room where she turns him or her over to receivers and finishes the chart. Then she returns to the OR to prepare for the next patient. She estimates she's performed this ballet at least 3,000 times.

Seifert, who is certified as both an operating room nurse and registered nurse first assistant, says that the work can be so stressful that at times she wonders why she does it. "But then a family member seeks you out to thank you and show their appreciation and you think, maybe I won't quit today," she says. In addition to patient feedback, another high is seeing "the new staff you've taken under your wing start to turn into butterflies."

The greatest part of her job, Seifert says, is seeing quick results, working with smart people, and being part of the aesthetics of operating. The human body fascinates her. Perhaps the greatest plus is how much what she does, matters. "You get a phone call from the emergency room that an aneurysm is ready to burst and you hustle to the OR. You help the surgeon get a chest opened fast and control the aorta so the patient doesn't bleed to death. These are true saves that require the utmost in teamwork, and no one could have done them alone."

Sometimes, of course, the patient isn't saved. Sometimes, when a patient dies on the OR table, Seifert sees that the patient is cleaned and moved to a quiet room. Then she takes the family in to see their loved one. "I never cover the head and I make a point of holding the patient's hand and stroking the forehead to signal that it's okay for them to touch. Seifert takes her cue from the family; if they want her to stay with them, she does. She

"In the OR, you need to make immediate decisions. The status of patients changes quickly and confident people are needed to make fast decisions and deliver fast, accurate assessments."

Patricia Seifert, RN, MSN, CRNFA, FAAN

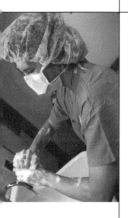

also calls for a religious counselor upon request. "You can't make death a happy occasion but you can at least help people begin the grieving process," she says.

Like other nurses, those who work in the OR need to work with the demands of administrators. "Of all the departments in a hospital, the OR makes the most money. But we also spend the most money, so administrators are interested in us," she says. "You need to talk their language to get what you want. You need to show them the value of capital purchases like a laser, drill or saw, for example." Seifert invites her administrators to watch surgery. "Sometimes I still have to fight for a request, but at least they'll have a mental picture of what I was talking about," she says.

Since Seifert began in the OR, technology and refinement of procedures has made recovery time incredibly faster. Patients have also become savvier because of the Internet. "In the old days, we were the only ones who taught patients. Now with all the other sources available we have to help them separate the wheat from the chaff."

Seifert sees a bright future for OR nurses with a myriad of opportunities. "Our skills are in big demand from surgical centers, resource management, insurance companies, educational institutions and managed care."

PATIENT POINT OF VIEW

The patient's life is in the hands of the surgeon and surgical team, but it's usually the nurse who actually holds the hand of the patient as he or she floats off to sleep. And it's the nurse's comforting words the patients hear when they feel discomfort. Patients trust the OR nurses who hope to calm their anxiety and who bring humanity to the cold steel of an operating room.

Did you know?
AORN, the Association of periOperative Registered Nurses, was formally organized between 1949 and 1954, and is now composed of over 41,000 perioperative registered nurses in the U.S. and abroad.

fast facts

What do you need?

o   Ability to interact well with all kinds of people in different situations
o   Emotional stability to cope with human suffering and frequent emergencies
o   Physical strength and stamina to position patients and transport equipment, and stand for hours on end at an operating table
o   Sense of humor

What's it take?

o   A current license as a Registered Nurse (RN)
o   BSN preferred, ADN usually sufficient for entry level
o   Post-graduate training in perioperative nursing

Where will you practice?

o   Hospital surgical departments
o   Ambulatory surgery centers
o   Clinics
o   Interventional suites
o   Physicians' offices
o   Physician office-based surgery

chapter twenty-six
psychiatric nurse

Psychiatric Nurse Checkpoint

Do you have an abiding interest in human behavior?

Would you enjoy advocating for those who have difficulty coping with their current life situation?

Do you believe that mental illness and emotional problems can be as life-threatening as medical disease?

If so, read on

A TRUE TALE

Although Ellen Mahoney, DNSc, RN, planned to major in English, after taking some anatomy and introductory nursing courses as a college freshman, she began to work her way towards a career in the healthcare field. "There was no single moment of enlightenment," the 50-year-old Mahoney laughs. "It was a continual thread that led me to nursing and my specialty as a career, and I've been doing it contentedly for 29 years."

After Mahoney graduated from Miseracordia College in Dallas, where she'd earned a BSN, she worked on a general medical-surgical unit at Massachusetts General Hospital. After another year in an intensive care unit, she moved to psychiatric nursing.

Mahoney later returned to school, taking two years to complete a psychiatric mental health nursing degree at Boston College. In May 2000, she added a doctorate in nursing science to her list of degrees. She'd been striving for it for eight years.

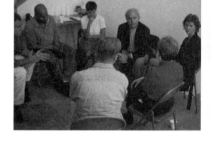

Psychiatric nursing is similar to general nursing in trying to meet the health needs of patients. But when the focus of care is mental health, Mahoney believes that technology doesn't play a very big role. She considers psychiatric nursing a misunderstood specialty. "Those who work in psychiatry identify it as a distinct arena but lay people don't perceive it as real nursing. One reason, of course, is that its practitioners don't wear uniforms or scrubs. Another is that the facilities we work in are often not general hospitals."

A day in the life

For the past 12 years Mahoney, as a professor at the Catholic University of America School of Nursing, has been dealing with the emotional struggle of people trying to turn around their lives after an addiction. Each week she, along with a social worker or addiction counselor, co-leads outpatient group sessions of clients recovering from overuse of alcohol or drugs. Referred by

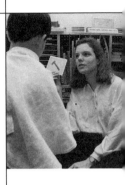

their primary care provider, the courts, or an attorney, 12 to 16 members come for a one-and-a-half or two-hour evening session. "They do this on average for a year. Typically most are fully committed to recovery and come regularly," Mahoney says.

Often, the attendees are at different points in their recovery. The group discusses what the week of each of the participants has been like, what if anything they have done to sabotage their recovery or to support it, and what other meetings they've attended. In the second hour the group focuses on a particular problem or person.

Mahoney gets to know them but they don't become friends, in order to honor intentional therapeutic professional boundaries. She facilitates patients giving each other feedback but does not offer her advice, treatment, or recommendations in these sessions. Mahoney acknowledges a high amount of recidivism among her clientele but insists that mental illness and addiction are "no different from any other chronic illness." She believes that some people are born with genetic predisposition to addiction but that personal qualities and the environment can nurture or regulate their propensity to give in to it.

Mahoney also teaches both graduate and undergraduate mental health courses, bringing students to the hospital for clinical rotations.

Mahoney holds two certifications: one for addictions nursing and one for clinical specialist in psychiatric mental health nursing. She recalls when she first started out, a man showed up in the acute detoxification center fifteen times in one year and she got to know him and his difficult battle with alcohol. Years later, after she'd moved to another treatment area, she saw him again and learned he'd been sober for six months. It's episodes like these that continue to make her feel wonderful about her career choice.

"You work largely in autonomous practice settings like clinics, group homes, community health centers and home care, which lends itself to the independent initiative of the nurse."

Ellen Mahoney, DNSc, RN

Profiling the job

Seeing patients regain their footing is fulfilling for Mahoney. "The 'biological piece' is fascinating, and the variety of opportunities psychiatric nursing affords the practitioner is fortuitous," she says. Working largely in autonomous practice settings such as clinics, group homes, community health centers and home care, she feels, lends itself to the independent initiative of the nurse. And it's very different from inpatient psychiatric units, where patients are sometimes restrained.

In hospitals, Mahoney has been tussled around by patients and has had to summon help. She knows how to hold patients and get them to the floor without harming them. "There's not a psychiatric nurse who hasn't had to wrestle someone at one time or another," she says. "It's not something I want to happen but when it does, I don't get upset."

Through the years, Mahoney has seen many who have attempted suicide, but she has never lost a patient in her direct care. However, she does know of former patients who have killed themselves and says she is "touched by their anguish. People often die of their addiction. It might not be as dramatic as a suicide but these are chemicals that can have deadly consequences."

The work is challenging, she admits. "It's not like when people go in for surgery and have an immediate change. Here you're in it for the long run. Behavioral changes take a long time and if you see patients for three to four days in the hospital you might never see what they accomplish outside. It's dispiriting to keep putting in and giving when you rarely see the pay-back." In group practice, she says, you see much more return on your investment.

The field of psychiatric nursing is becoming increasingly attractive to young nurses. Part of the attraction is due to the ever greater expanse of biological information in the field and the realization that professionals get involved in subjects such as neuroanatomy and physiology. Another possible attraction is the multitude of new and effective pharmacologic agents available that work against disorders.

At the same time, resources are dwindling, leading to shorter hospital stays. "Unfortunately, our patients are sicker when they arrive and when they leave. Treatment programs used to take one-and-a-half years. Now, after 30 days, we might mainstream them without support. For many of these people, unfortunately, the systems in place are setting them up to fail. This leads to a situation when society bears the burden of their bizarre or desperate behavior. Many of these patients also have a chronic medical condition which goes largely unmanaged."

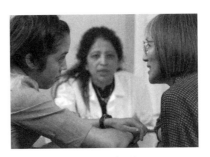

Mahoney predicts that tighter money may ultimately result in more innovative approaches, such as mobile treatment on the street. That is, increasingly healthcare professionals will drive around in vans and tend to people with schizophrenia, bipolar disorder, major depression, obsessive-compulsive disorder, and severe anxiety disorders. "Students in progressive assertive treatment centers are taking the treatment where it needs to go — to the patient under the bridge."

The greatest career joy for Mahoney is recognizing that if treatment is successful it's because of her and her colleagues. "A machine or physical intervention didn't do that. It means you have learned how to use yourself in a helpful way."

PATIENT POINT OF VIEW
One evening on the psychiatric unit of the hospital a very sick woman in seclusion was yelling for hours. Every time anyone came toward her, she became violent. One determined nurse was set on helping her. As the evening wore on this nurse talked to her from a distance and then edged closer and closer until they were finally next to each other. The hostility had leeched away and the woman was able to nestle down and go to sleep for the night.

>>> fast facts

What do you need?
- Psychological and physical stamina
- Medical skills
- Special interest in psychopharmacology and counseling
- Ability to deal with uncooperative or difficult/dangerous clients

What's it take?
- A current license as a Registered Nurse (RN)
- BSN preferred, ADN usually sufficient for entry level
- Certification as a psychiatric mental health nurse

Where will you practice?
- Hospitals
- Outpatient facilities
- Health departments
- Long-term care centers

1 Brink, Susan. "For severe mental illness, a higher profile and new hope". US News Online. Dec. 20 1999.
http://www.usnews.com/usnews/issue/991220/nycu/mental/htm

chapter twenty-seven

rehabilitation nurse

A TRUE TALE

Judy DiFilippo, RN, knew she would be a nurse from the time she was in third grade. That was when she read the Cherry Ames children's book on nursing. In high school she worked as a candy striper and a nurse's aide. Her mother wanted to be a nurse when she was young, but DiFilippo's grandfather forbade it. DiFilippo resolved to become a nurse for both of them.

**Rehabilitation
Nurse
Checkpoint**

Do you enjoy managing complex medical issues?

Would you like to be involved with a large number of patients?

Would you find it very satisfying to help someone achieve maximal independence?

If so, read on

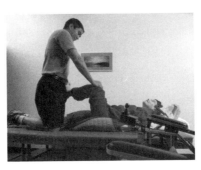

Her nursing skills have taken her all over the country. After graduation in 1969 from St. Xavier University, a small women's college in Chicago, she began work as an orthopedic neuro-surgical nurse. Shortly after, she began teaching in a three-year nursing program. In 1974 she returned to school for a master's degree in rehabilitative nursing.

This served her quite well when, several years later, master's degree in hand, DiFilippo returned to the classroom. This time, though, it was she who was the teacher. "Among other things, I taught nursing students the basics and the specifics. From how to move patients in bed to how to promote independence in someone who's had a stroke. I took what I'd learned in rehabilitation nursing and incorporated it into my teaching," the 53-year-old says. But after some time, she began to miss hands-on nursing. That's when she became a clinical specialist in the rehabilitation unit of Mercy Hospital in Chicago. While there, she developed an occupational nursing rehabilitation program to help get injured workers back on the job sooner.

A day in the life

DiFilippo is currently working as a manager of clinical operations for the adult rehabilitation unit at Advocate Christ Medical Center in Oak Lawn, Illinois. The 37-bed unit provides rehabilitation programs for patients with brain and spinal cord injury, and general rehabilitation problems — usually neurological or orthopedic in nature. The rehabilitation nurses on the unit typically have six patients for whom they coordinate care and provide

Did you know?
It is estimated
that savings
in long-term
disability costs
range from
$1 billion to
$2 billion
annually when
rehabilitation
is used. That's
because rehabil-
itation often
halts the pro-
gression of pri-
mary and
secondary
disabilities, so
that people
can return to
their jobs.[1]

medication and treatments. "Instead of focusing on illness, we focus on our patients' abilities," she says. "We evaluate their ability to cope with the effects of their illnesses." After therapy she encourages her patients to prac- tice the skills they learned. The goal is to get them to increase their skills and level of endurance so that they can make a successful transition at home.

And getting patients home is something that's happening more quickly these days, perhaps due to cost constraints and other factors. "Twenty years ago people would stay in a hospital four to six months for a spinal cord injury, but now they go home in weeks. Then again, we may have made them a bit more dependent on us than they should have been," says DiFilippo.

Profiling the job

The support team DiFilippo puts together is comprised of a psychologist, social service practitioner, recreational therapist, physical therapist, occupa- tional therapist, speech pathologist and nurses from various disciplines. This team helps patients return to an optimum level of functioning. An important discussion DiFilippo always schedules with her patients is the one concerning how they think their new loss of skills will affect their lives when they return home. Many are intensely angry about what has happened to them and they need to deal with their feelings. This is a major part of the rehabilita- tion process, and like other members of the team, DiFilippo is always a willing listener.

"In rehabilitation, people are with you for a much longer period of time than they are with a general-care nurse. As a result, you develop real relationships with them and can be helpful as they cope with the new adjustments to their lives."

After DiFilippo's patients are treated in the hospital, they are transitioned to outpatient facilities or to the home to receive home health services. "It is called rehabilitation without walls," she says. With the emergence of more portable equipment and specialized skills to bring to the patient, she feels that home rehabilita- tion can only increasingly get better.

DiFilippo reflects on one of her former patients, a violinist with the Chicago Symphony Orchestra. Years ago, the man came into the hospital unable to move. After a year of rehabilitation he went back to playing his violin, she says. "It's watching this man progress as he did, and knowing I played a role in his progress, that keeps me committed. I'm in a great specialty of nursing. The huge changes in functionality of our patients is a tremendous payback."

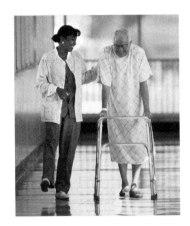

"Instead of focusing on the illness, rehabilitation focuses on the patient's abilities and how he or she is adapting to the disability or the effects of chronic illness."

Judy DiFilippo, RN

PATIENT POINT OF VIEW

Nurses are often the stopgap needed to ensure adequate care, potentially to the disabled patient. They respond to the patient's needs as well as his or her family experiencing them. Sometimes, families coping with life-changing circumstances need education to learn to manage the wide range of challenges they and their loved one will face. Rehabilitation nurses provide an integrated approach to medical, vocational, educational, environmental and spiritual needs. They not only act as caregivers but also as coordinators and case managers, bringing together specialists to help people achieve optimal functionality and independence.

fast facts

What do you need?

o Either of the following:
  - Two or more years of practice in rehabilitation
  - One or more year of practice in rehabilitation combined with one year of advanced study in nursing
o An RN with a Certified Rehabilitation Registered Nurse (CRRN) and a master's degree or doctorate in nursing can earn certification as a CRRN-Advanced (CRRN-A)
o Fifteen classroom hours or at least 15 contract hours in the core content of rehabilitation nursing

What's it take?

o A current license as a Registered Nurse (RN)
o A certification examination in rehabilitation nursing
o BSN preferred, ADN usually sufficient for entry level

Where will you practice?

o Hospitals
o Comprehensive inpatient rehabilitation units
o Sub-acute facilities
o Long-term care facilities
o Home healthcare agencies
o Skilled nursing facilities
o Clinics
o Community and governmental agencies
o Insurance companies
o Health maintenance organizations
o Schools and universities
o Outpatient rehabilitation facilities

Other opportunities

o Administrator
o Admissions liaison
o Case manager
o Clinical nurse specialist
o Researcher
o Staff nurse
o Educator

---

1 Association of Rehabilitative Nurses. "The Appropriate Inclusion of Rehabilitation Nurses Wherever Rehabilitation is Provided". http://www.rehabnurse.org/resources00/position/pappropr.htm

research nurse

A TRUE TALE

Twenty-four year old Melissa Allan, RN, BSN, grew up in a family of nurses. Her mother, older sister and brother are all members of the profession. When she started as a registered nurse on the progressive care unit at Florida South Hospital, Allan looked after patients recovering from open heart surgery. The technology, combined with the intricate workings of the heart itself, fascinated her. "I wanted to learn more about the heart and about cardiovascular research altogether," she says. After a preceptorship in which she followed a research nurse around, Allan was convinced she'd found her calling.

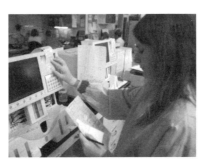

A day in the life

A typical day for Allan in the Cardiovascular Research Department begins at 6:00am and finishes at 3:00pm. Her job is to screen patients for one of the 25 or so clinical trials taking place. Her first task is to review the charts of prospective entrants. If they fit the required protocol, she then approaches the patient.

Getting patients to participate in a clinical trial is extremely involved and requires a great deal of time and commitment on everyone's part. It is, after all, asking someone to opt for an untried treatment as opposed to one that has been used for years. So, it's essential that patients understand fully all that is required of them and what the benefits are to them. First, Allan explains the project fully. Then she discusses the risks and benefits with the patient. She also discusses the probability that the new treatment may be a better alternative to what is currently available, and that participants in the trial may receive any number of potential therapies being studied and the risks of each. If they agree to participate, they must sign an informed consent. Most of the patients she queries agree to participate. But some decline because they "don't want to be a guinea pig," she says. Those who do participate often do so because of the benefits to society that research brings. Others are looking for a better, easier or more effective treatment.

Research Nurse Checkpoint

Do you have an intense thirst for cutting-edge knowledge?

Are you detail-oriented and capable of doing a large amount of paperwork?

Do you desire autonomy and responsibility to be in charge of many things at once?

If so, read on

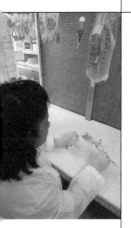

Once the participants are enrolled in the study, Allan brings each one to the lab with the physician to review the procedure step-by-step to ensure it follows the protocol. She typically reviews the progress of 50 to 60 patients a day. Because she has so many protocols to keep track of, she makes little five-by-seven "reminder cards" listing inclusion and exclusion criteria for each program. She carries 20 of these cards on a ring like a key chain.

Allan works with three research coordinators and an assistant. An administrator, who is the department supervisor, handles the legal and regulatory aspects of screening and makes arrangements with the various research sponsors whose medicines and procedures are tested. Responsibilities include insuring prospective patient recruitment, protocol compliance, proper handling of investigational drugs and supplies, patient monitoring, reporting and study completion. Practicing in a research environment demands a high level of sophistication in patient care skills, new technology and regulation. What Allan likes most is the environment in which she works and the cutting-edge knowledge she feels her co-workers possess. "During orientation I sat in a catheterization lab to watch an angiogram being performed. It was fascinating," she says. She also enjoys her contact with ancillary departments. "I generally have access to everyone and enjoy interacting regularly with physicians, patients and surgical technicians," she says. "But I also like having the ability to practice great autonomy – in a sense I am like an independent agent."

"A lot of people don't know what being a research nurse entails," Allan admits.
"It's not just petri dishes in a lab. There's often a lot more patient contact than with regular patient care."

Profiling the job

Some of the clinical trials require following patients for 24 hours; others demand vigilance for up to five years. Patients generally like this, says Allan, because as a result they are monitored more closely. "We call them on the phone and make sure they are taking their medication and that they return for follow-up tests. Many of them find great security in knowing they 'belong to us' for the length of the study."

PATIENT POINT OF VIEW

Depending on the scope of the protocol, a patient's involvement with a research nurse can range from minimal to extensive. Research nurses are a liaison between the patient and the investigating team. They explain the actual procedure and review the benefits and risks with the patient. The research nurse follows the patient — sometimes briefly, other times for years — in an effort to assure the patient's long-term health status and adherence to study requirements. In this age of faceless medicine, patients in clinical trials become far more than a case number, and much of this is due to the research nurse's intervention.

fast facts

What do you need?
- Strong observation and analytical skills
- An ability to concentrate on details
- Grant writing experience may be helpful

What's it take?
- A Bachelor of Science in Nursing (BSN)
- A master's degree
- Advanced nursing research may require a PhD

Where will you practice?
- Pharmaceutical companies
- Contract research organizations
- Teaching and university hospitals
- Educational institutions
- Temporary technical placement agencies

chapter twenty-nine
school nurse

School Nurse Checkpoint

Do you like a school environment?

Is it of prime importance to have "normal" hours and summers off?

Do you enjoy being around healthy children?

If so, read on

A TRUE TALE

At 26, Sue Sherman, RN, MS, quit her job as a bank teller to return to school. She'd always had an interest in nursing — and after years of handling money, she was convinced she'd rather be "handling" people. She selected a local community college 50 miles north of Albany, New York for its two-year RN course. In 1985 she began her nursing career in a family practice office. Subsequently, she signed on with an agency as a nurse for developmentally disabled adults.

Two years ago she went back to school again — this time as the nurse in a local high school. Most of Sherman's days are now taken up with first aid and minor illnesses, but she deals with some of the student's social issues as well.

A day in the life

Sherman arrives at school by 7:45am and leaves at 3:15pm. Most, but far from all, of her students have general complaints. Pre-suicidal thoughts and violence have been on the minds of a few, she says, and she has been on the front lines of several unwanted pregnancies. She also sees head and athletic injuries and seizures. In the past two years, two students have died: one from bacterial meningitis and the other in a car crash.

Sherman is in charge of all the students' sports physicals (working with a school physician who comes in three times a year) for which she screens hearing and vision. If it is determined that a student needs glasses, Sherman works with the school counselor and social service worker to make certain that the student obtains them. As a school nurse, she automatically serves as a team member of the school's emergency plan.

Sometimes her job involves alerting an unknowing teacher to a child's medical condition. "One teacher wasn't allowing a diabetic to leave the room because she was unaware of his disease," says Sherman. "We have a social worker that comes to our school. Programs that she offers, and in which I am happy to get involved, include issues of sexually transmitted diseases, drugs and alcohol. Our wellness programs are equally popular and just as important" she says. These include nutrition, exercise, weight management, and smoking cessation.

Profiling the job

When Sherman detects something she believes needs follow-up, such as potential scoliosis or even an abnormal mole, she suggests to the student and his or her parents that the child see a physician. Often the family's insurance, or lack of it, complicates which physician is available to them, a major frustration to a school nurse — who will step in and do everything to try to help.

That kind of frustration, in addition to less than stellar pay, are the negatives to the job. The positives, however, outweigh them. "There's great flexibility and autonomy, terrific hours and cooperation from the kids and their parents," she says. "Working the school calendar with summers off is a big plus." Students refer to her as Mrs. Sherman and she doesn't wear a uniform. "My own kids often stop in and say 'hi'," she adds. "It's reassuring to see how many teenagers are like my own in some ways, but in other ways, it's nice to see that there's such variety out there."

PATIENT POINT OF VIEW

I'm pretty healthy and don't go to the nurse much. But whenever I pass her in the hall or go to her office, she knows my name and asks how I'm doing. She knows I find it hard to see the blackboard and to concentrate, so she's worked with my teachers to allow me to sit where it's best for me to learn. My parents think she's overcautious because she sends kids home when they've got a cold but that's because my parents only have me and my sister to worry about. The school nurse has to worry about everyone.

Andrew, 8th grade, New York

"Working with teenagers can be tough. You've got to take the time to get to know them. Sometimes you've got to utilize every resource available to solve the puzzles they present."

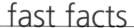

fast facts

What do you need?

○ To practice in accordance with current standards as identified by the National Association of School Nurses

○ A 250-question, four-hour exam for NCSN certification

○ Certain counseling skills may be required

What's it take?

○ A current license as a Registered Nurse (RN)

○ A Bachelor of Science in Nursing (BSN) in some states

○ NCSN certification (provides formal recognition of basic school nursing knowledge) may be required

Where will you practice?

○ School systems

○ County health departments

○ State health departments

Content

urology nurse

A TRUE TALE

Donna Brassil, MA, RN, CURN, comes from a family of nurses. Her mother and several of her aunts are in the profession. Growing up in Queens, New York, she helped nurse sick relatives and experienced firsthand what illness can do to people and their families. That, combined with the fact that Brassil has a nurturing personality by nature, sealed her choice of profession.

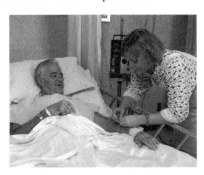

More than 20 years ago during nursing school at SUNY, Downstate Medical Center in New York, a clinical rotation in urology convinced her that this field "was a lot more than little old men with Foley catheters." Armed with a BSN degree, she joined the urology unit of New York University Medical Center 22 years ago as a staff nurse.

Her role as a staff nurse called for a variety of responsibilities, such as taking vital signs and treating pre- and post-operative conditions. Patient education was a vital part, too, Brassil recalls. In addition to general nursing skills, urologic nurses must understand urodynamics, infectious diseases, renal pathophysiology, as well as urologic pathophysiology, and sexual dysfunction.

Later, Brassil was elevated to head nurse on the urology unit. In this capacity, her role shifted away from patient care to staff management. "Creating an environment to foster the staff's growth and development was my number one priority," she remarks. "I helped my staff understand the importance of patient education and worked towards this end so that all patients in their care would benefit."

After a six-year stint, Brassil became Director of Nursing for all surgical services at the hospital. She was responsible for all surgical departments including urology, gynecology, neurology, neurosurgery, orthopedics, plastic and general surgery, as well as cardiovascular and transplant. "I would say that my main charge in this position was to create and implement a team-building atmosphere and to encourage a leadership group that worked well with the staff and patients."

Urology Nurse Checkpoint

Are you intrigued by the renal system?

Are you comfortable talking about urologic conditions and sexual dysfunction?

Are you comfortable discussing "sensitive" issues with strangers?

If so, read on

However, Brassil soon missed patient care. This, and her fascination with nephrology, led her to a position that afforded her more time in this realm. Two years ago, she became Director of Clinical Trials for the Department of Urology at NYU, a position she still holds today. "To be an effective leader in the research area, one must have a strong clinical knowledge base that needs to begin at the roots of your first job as an RN," she says. By working in clinical trials, Brassil offers hope to patients by providing urologic treatment options that are otherwise not readily available.

Profiling the job

Today medicine can identify congenital anomalies that couldn't be classified years ago. This includes many associated with the field of urology. Even more gratifying to Brassil is to see many former patients return and "describe the improvement in the quality of their lives." In the urology unit, emotions run the gamut — humor, fear, embarrassment, grief. She tries to "read the patients" ahead of time to know how best to deal with them. "For example, someone who's an engineer or teacher tends to be detail-oriented, so with them I'm usually very detailed and statistical. I provide as much information as I think a patient can process. The more, the better, for all involved." She always shakes their hands and always spends as much time as a first-time patient needs. "Whatever the problem, it's always a worry to the patient. Urology is a more sensitive subject than most, since the very nature of it is so private. We recognize that and respect it."

"Erectile dysfunction and female sexual arousal disorder are being treated with regularity now because society is much more open about such issues," she says.

Since Brassil started in urology, the diagnostic tools have improved considerably. Today there are faster, less invasive procedures like Prostate Specific Antigen (PSA) tests, which help identify those with prostate cancer. Laparoscopy, for example, has turned major surgery into minor surgery so patients can be discharged sooner. Managed care has also mandated that the length of hospital stays be shortened. Now, more patients are treated in clinics and doctors' offices, rather than hospitals. And Brassil anticipates that in the future, there will be many more breakthrough choices and solutions for those with urologic erectile cancers, dysfunction, urinary incontinence and female sexual arousal disorder. Brassil says one of the ways for nurses to

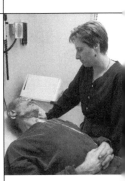

keep current is to join a nursing specialty organization. "Being a member of the Society of Urologic Nurses and Associates has provided me with a forum in which to gain further education and an opportunity to gain support from my peers. For me, this has been invaluable."

PATIENT POINT OF VIEW

Usually a diagnosis of prostate cancer comes just at mid-life, when a man is facing doubts about his manliness as well as his future. Couple that with the fear of cancer itself, and you've got the ingredients for a frightened and depressed patient. Once a diagnosis is confirmed, there's the need to determine which treatment to pursue – surgery, chemotherapy, radiation or hormone therapy. Before being diagnosed, most men knew nothing about prostate cancer, so patient education and counseling are very important. Many who have gone through it credit a sympathetic and compassionate nurse with "saving their lives" in more ways than one.

fast facts

What do you need?
- Fifty continuing education (CE) contact hours per year
- Thirty-six CE hours in study pertinent to the field of urology
- At least 800 hours of practice during the previous three years in order to be eligible for re-certification

What's it take?
- BSN preferred, ADN usually sufficient for entry level
- Current certification by CBUNA is preferable
- A current license for RN/LPN/NP

Where will you practice?
- Hospitals
- Clinics
- Inpatient/outpatient facilities
- Physicians' offices

chapter thirty-one
veteran's affairs nurse

**VA Nurse
Checkpoint**

Do you have a
strong sense of
community?

Do you want
to lock in
benefits and
a set schedule
that precludes
working
holidays?

Would you be
interested in
following
the health of
your patients
long term?

If so, read on

A TRUE TALE

Getting into the Veterans arena was a matter of luck for Maureen Furnari, RN. A girlfriend was in charge of the operating room (OR) at a Veteran's Affairs (VA) hospital and was seeking new nurses just at the time Furnari, armed with a BSN from Bellevue School of Nursing, was seeking a new job.

When she started at Brooklyn Veterans Hospital, Furnari worked as a scrub nurse in the OR. Then she moved into urology as both a scrub and circulating nurse. The type of nursing care rendered in the VA hospital, she says, was similar to what she had done in other hospitals, but the population was different. "These guys, and most of the vets here are guys, can be very funny. They're grateful for anything you do for them," she says. "They don't expect anything, which sure is different from the

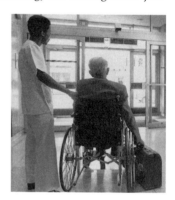

outside world, where most people can be quite demanding." Furnari and some of her nursing associates in veteran's care feel that these patients are more compliant than the ones you'll find in a general hospital. "As military and ex-military personnel, they're used to taking orders from senior officers, and if you tell them to do something that's important for their health, they usually will," she says.

The "guys" increasingly include women these days, with an age range from 20 to 99 years. The facility is open to active duty servicemen and service-women, and to any veteran with an identification card or the appropriate discharge papers. All are treated the same "whether they're a prisoner of war or a cook in the Army," says Furnari. "In my clinic it's first come, first served."

Profiling the job

The VA facility offers comprehensive healthcare services from prescription eyeglasses to liver transplants. The services are dispensed equally to all, but what recipients pay for those services depends on their position in or service to the Army, Navy, Air Force or Marines. Patients with conditions stemming from injuries sustained during service pay nothing, while other veterans must pay at least something. Furnari estimates that 10 percent of patients have private insurance. Technically, the facility is open from 9:00am to 3:00pm, but Furnari regularly opens her doors at 7:30am in order to treat some of the people that have to go to work.

But the broad spectrum and quality of care offered to veterans, Furnari feels, is sometimes overlooked. "VA medical care doesn't always get the notoriety it deserves," she says. With over 172 hospitals, the VA is the world's largest organized healthcare system — and it has the largest nursing service. This works well because nurses can network within the system — calling any hospital in any state for advice on unusual cases. One opportunity in this field not found elsewhere is the ability to follow patients for years. That's because they keep coming back for treatment of medical problems. The hospital's population includes long-term chronic hospital-housed patients and those who come in for annual checkups. Furnari adds that seeing patients over the years is an excellent opportunity for the medical researchers, too. In fact, the VA health system is second only to the NIH in research.

Furnari says she earns around 20 percent less than she would in the outside world, but she enjoys five weeks of vacation time and doesn't work holidays or weekends.

A day in the life
On a typical day Furnari, who is 41, will see 12 to 20 patients for outpatient ambulatory procedures such as cystoscopies or prostate biopsies. She counsels, consoles, and answers batteries of questions. Perhaps once a week, she informs a patient of a life-threatening condition.

When patients are ready to go home, Furnari gives them their discharge instructions. She also gives patients the unit's phone number and urges them to call at any time. Elderly patients may forget many details of what the nurse tells them once they have walked out the door. Recognizing this, she welcomes family members' questions or phone calls. In fact, she encourages both.

Did you know?
With 172 hospitals, the VA is the largest organized healthcare system in the world with the largest nursing service. A distinct advantage is that nurses can network through the system.

"Nurses can network through the large system — and nurses can transfer from one VA hospital to another without loss of benefits. Usually, our population is made up of people with chronic problems, so when we say goodbye, we know — and they do too — that we'll probably be seeing them again," she says.

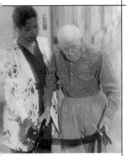

Conditions at the VA have improved dramatically since Furnari arrived. "We've got new equipment arriving daily and we're doing less surgery because there's more effective results with medicine available."

PATIENT POINT OF VIEW

Today's veterans may not be esteemed the way those who served their country in earlier times and past wars have been, but in the VA hospitals every serviceman and servicewoman is a time-honored guest. The nurses only reinforce this by offering technical skill, comfort and support, and an understanding of what being in the Armed Forces means.

>>> # fast facts

What do you need?
- Valid citizenship of the United States
- To be proficient in spoken and written English
- Experience as a Graduate Nurse Technician (GNT), Nurse Technician Pending Graduation

What's it take?
- Associate degree or diploma in nursing
- Baccalaureate degree in nursing from NLNAC/CCNE-accredited program
- A current license as a Registered Nurse (RN)

Where will you practice?
- Hospitals
- VA Homes
- Nursing homes
- Private residences

the nurse in
management

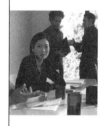

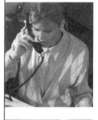

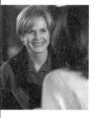

managing a health center & the value of an MBA

Eleven years ago, the Columbia University School of Nursing faculty began studying scholarly practices of its specialties to determine what procedures offered the best care for patients and were most cost-efficient to deliver. In 1994, it seeded pioneer practices where several faculty members could work together at various sites around New York City. The result was the formation of CAPNA (Columbia Advanced Practice Nurse Associates), a primary care practice where all providers are advanced practice nurses.

By Linda Gibbs, RN, MBA, Assistant Dean of Practice Development, Columbia University School of Nursing

As the Assistant Dean of Practice Development for Columbia University School of Nursing, I am responsible for all non-clinical aspects of our two CAPNA practices, one at the Columbia hospital campus and an additional site in midtown Manhattan. As an RN with an MBA, my responsibilities include strategic planning, reimbursement, operational streamlining and regulatory compliance. The skills I obtained through my advanced degree in business have been essential for my job.

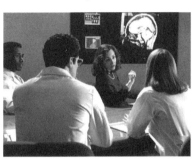

As the CAPNA practice grows, strategic planning becomes increasingly important. One area in particular that I'm interested in is how we bring value to our patients, and in maintaining patient satisfaction while increasing our practice capacity. Our three advanced practice nurses (APNs), all of whom have master's degrees, diagnose and treat patients and can write prescriptions as needed. We schedule considerably longer visits than most primary care physicians do because our focus is on providing more education. If there is a need for a specialist we refer patients to Columbia physicians. Mostly our APNs are involved in such primary care needs as normal annual physicals, questions about menopause, asthma, diabetes and nutrition. We evaluate and treat acute, episodic and chronic disease, take medical, family, and psychosocial histories, develop and implement therapeutic regimens, and emphasize prevention. The APNs also have admitting privileges at the Columbia-Presbyterian Center of New York Presbyterian Hospital.

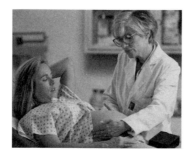

Studies show that at least 80 percent of primary care office visits can be managed equally well by either primary care physicians or APNs. They have also shown that when APNs perform a large percent of the procedures, it is a very cost-effective method of providing care. Additionally, APNs tend to score higher on patient satisfaction surveys than physicians do. Surveys show that patients treated by advanced practice nurses were more likely to stick with their provider's care than those treated by physicians, and they preferred an APN's personal manner and time spent with the patient.

Around 75 percent of our patients are on a commercial insurance plan. CAPNA participates in 11 insurance plans and also accepts Medicaid/ Medicare. As a result, we address reimbursement issues on a daily basis. We analyze contracted fee and reimbursement agreements and evaluate account receivables. Additionally, we try to minimize our operating costs associated with inventory control and overhead.

Regulatory compliance is another area where a lot of analytical time is spent. Because each state addresses advanced practice nurses differently, understanding and keeping up with the federal and state regulations that allow APNs to practice is essential. I also examine how new regulations will effect our practice. For example, the Health Care Information Portability Accountability Act (HIPAA) will certainly impact CAPNA. At present, we are examining how this legislation will affect the electronic transfer of information from practice sites.

Today, in the United States, there are increasing opportunities in senior decision-making positions for all healthcare practitioners with advanced business degrees. Nurses with expertise in finance, law, human resources and computer science have inordinate opportunities to develop better systems for healthcare administration and delivery. They can work, for example, in industry, administrative positions, insurance, education, for third parties and in government. While their work is business-oriented, it still profoundly impacts the broad healthcare delivery system and, of course, the lives of patients.

Linda Gibbs has been a Healthcare Consultant at PricewaterhouseCoopers LLC in New York. There she worked on strategic planning projects, conducted research on industry trends and formulated reports on competitive data. Before that, Mrs. Gibbs had been a Financial Planning Associate in a Medicaid Assistance Program (MAP). At MAP she analyzed budgets, performed statistical analysis of rates and savings and studied the prospective revenues for payers under Medicaid Managed Care. She has performed utilization review for the Health Insurance Plan of New York and was an emergency room nurse at Mount Sinai Hospital in New York City for three years. Mrs. Gibbs earned an MBA from Columbia Business School and a BSN from the University of Michigan in Ann Arbor. She is deeply involved in educating the public and healthcare community about nurse practitioners and how they fit into the primary care model.

By Harriet
Feldman,
PhD, RN, FAAN,
Dean and
Professor,
Lienhard School
of Nursing,
Pace University

the nurse in management
leadership goals and general administration issues

When I was growing up and considering nursing as a profession, I always imagined I'd be a bedside nurse. Indeed, I started off as a staff nurse and loved it, but soon moved into education and finally, as a fluke, I tried out administration. I never imagined I'd stay to be an organizer, administrator, writer, and change agent, but life has taken me here — and I'm very happy it has. Many administrators share skills with clinical practitioners, but running the show requires other abilities as well. I've tried to spell out the ones I consider most important.

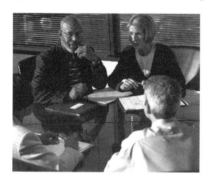

First of all, the responsibility that goes along with being an administrator means you need to understand how to work closely and well with other people. Of course that's a requirement in all nursing roles; however, sometimes it can take you down a difficult road. Once, a group of my nursing students objected to the teaching style, attitude and competence of a new faculty member I'd hired. I met with small groups of them and with other faculty members and listened to their concerns. From what they said, I could see that this teacher's behavior would adversely affect their learning. I had to take the hard but necessary step of discharging the new faculty member. In other words: the buck stops here.

To be an effective administrator you need to be a leader with a vision for the future. A while ago I attended a national meeting where healthcare changes were discussed, and I quickly realized how traditional our curriculum was. It focused mainly on acute care for hospitalized patients. This, I felt, did not address the community's needs, as an increasing number of people are being treated at home and through clinics and outside programs. I brought this message back to our campus and ultimately motivated the faculty to dramatically change the curriculum to focus on primary healthcare both inside and outside of the hospital setting. As a learning experience, the faculty brought students to the Henry Street Settlement in lower Manhattan, a center that provides services to a lower-income and sometimes

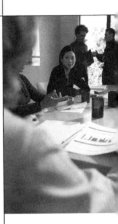

deeply disadvantaged community. Here the students learned that providing for the healthcare and the needs of a community is much more than providing medical treatments.

As a leader or administrator you need to have a passion for developing and mentoring others. I have relied on mentors to get where I am today. After being in nursing for 35 years and a dean for the past 14, I'm now interested in succession planning, which means developing people to carry out areas of leadership by helping them follow their own focus and direction. For example, I chair the mentoring committee of the American Association of Colleges of Nursing, which matches new deans with more seasoned ones who know how to manage the ropes of higher education and are knowledgeable about budgets, strategic planning, and other current issues.

Other requirements of a quality leader are a strong sense of self and an ability to separate yourself as a person from the job you do. Though you may be "friends" with a co-worker, you have to realize that when you make a tough decision it's in the capacity of administrator, not friend. Flexibility is also important. Sometimes you've got to compromise and sometimes you have to give in, even when you're loathe to do so, because it's for the greater good.

You also need to be comfortable with the notion of risk-taking. Of course, you have to evaluate risks to know which ones are "safe," and be aware that sometimes taking risks puts you in the hot seat. I took a big risk shortly after coming to Pace University. In less than a year I dramatically changed the organizational structure of the School of Nursing. I shifted around people's responsibilities and in doing so, ultimately gave faculty and staff greater input into decisions. As a result, people found themselves working harder and being more accountable for their actions. Inevitably, there were negative reactions from some, which challenged me to think about my leadership style and how to best facilitate change. But on the whole, the positions and people in them adapted fairly quickly.

There is also a need to focus on continuous quality improvement. Nurses — all nurses — always strive to learn and grow because the world around us is ever-changing. As professionals, we need to be mindful of keeping pace and moving agendas forward; we can't stay fixed and expect to survive. Now more than ever before, professional accrediting groups insist that we be acutely aware of quality improvement and responsive to standards that change with time. This holds true for both the clinical and educational settings. Quality care at a reasonable cost is the goal in clinical settings and quality education at a reasonable cost is the goal of higher education.

A leader needs good listening skills. This lets others know that you have confidence and are interested in them, and that their ideas are worthy and important. Each person brings a unique point of view to an issue and, while we may not always agree, it is important that we respect our differences. This is also very important in the nurse-patient relationship. Good listening also means that you're fully present and focused on what your colleagues have to say.

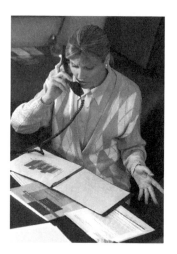

Finally, I must say this: A great sense of humor may well be your greatest asset. It also makes you more approachable and it makes work less boring. I just finished reading a management guide about how to make the work place "nicer." More than half of our time awake is spent at work, so why not bring a sunny disposition there? The author of the book noted that people can choose the attitude they bring to the work setting. A positive attitude generates good will and energy among your "customers," which in the case of an educational setting are our students and those for whom they care.

Creating a perfect environment where professionals can do the best job isn't always possible, but it's a worthy goal. One way to accomplish this goal is to set clear standards and gain acceptance from those professionals doing the grassroots work. Another way is being supportive of the people who work with you and encouraging them to grow. One area I've been successful with is developing faculty scholarship, particularly with respect to research. It is rewarding to see people who have conducted innumerable hours of research finally publish their results in a respected nursing journal.

People sometimes ask me if I miss the "nursing" part of nursing, but the truth is, I don't. I don't, because I'm doing it. Administration is just another way to practice nursing. It's different from clinical practice, but at the same time I'm helping to prepare the next generation of nurses with all the same motivations I had when I entered nursing as a young woman. Only now I can make a bigger impact on people's care by preparing other people to take care of patients. So, indirectly I'm caring for all of them.

Dr. Feldman received her PhD from New York University in research and theory development in nursing science and MS and BS degrees from Adelphi University. A specialist in the areas of pain perception and management, Dr. Feldman is a fellow of the American Academy of Nursing and has a certificate from the Harvard University Management Development program. Dr. Feldman is a noted author and co-author of more than 35 publications on research topics. She is co-founder of the journal Scholarly Inquiry for Nursing Practice *and is current editor of the journal* Nursing Leadership Forum. *Her most recent books are* Nurses in the Political Arena: The Public Face of Nursing, *co-authored with Dr. Sandra B. Lewenson,* Strategies for Nursing Leadership, *and* Nursing Leaders Speak Out, *all published by Springer. She is President of the Deans and Directors of Nursing in Greater New York and chair of the Mentoring Subcommittee of the American Association of Colleges of Nursing. For the past three years she has served as Chairperson of the University's Institutional Review Board.*

the value of an associate nursing degree

By Marilyn
Kaufmann,
PhD, RN,
Chair, Associate
Degree Nursing
Program,
Lakeshore
Technical
College

Nearly 50 years ago, an aspiring nurse had only one educational choice: the diploma program. At that point in time, students attended hospital-based or hospital-affiliated schools for three years to work as "student nurses." The eventual closing of these schools and a trend to college level training occurred. However, new opportunities for nursing careers opened up and prospective practitioners gained some additional choices.

Today's nurse has three different educational paths into nursing practice: diploma, baccalaureate degree (BSN) and associate degree (ADN). It should be noted, however, that fewer than 100 diploma schools remain in the U.S.

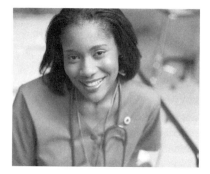

The BSN — a four-year degree offered mostly by standard colleges or universities — covers liberal arts as well as nursing skills, theory, research and management, and prepares the student for all professional aspects of nursing.

The two-year ADN focuses primarily on nursing's direct care giving skills. Because associate programs are shorter in duration than baccalaureate, the majority focus on direct nursing care subjects and are found at technical and community colleges. The ADN curricula includes courses such as anatomy and physiology, chemistry, psychology, microbiology, pharmacology and computer technology, as well as core medical — surgical, pediatric, obstetric, and mental health nursing. Some aspects of management, delegation and supervision are also taught as part of this degree program.

Some of my nursing colleagues and I are champions of the ADN because we believe that this degree remains an important pathway into nursing because of its flexibility and the limitless opportunities it provides. It's the first choice of the majority of nursing students entering the field for many reasons. First, if time is of the essence, an ADN allows you to take the RN exam sooner and find work more quickly. If your ultimate goal is hands-on nursing and direct patient care, an associate degree is all you need. Second, if finances are an issue, some students choose an ADN over a BSN because the cost of a four-year college can be prohibitive for them. Third, others choose to remain in the community in which they live, so attending a comunity college is the best option for them. Finally, those students who may be interested in testing the waters before committing to a nursing career find an ADN optimal because of its shorter time investment. Completion of an ADN may also allow the new nurse to begin practice to help finance future education in nursing.

Once you have completed your ADN studies, passed the RN exam and are ready to head into the job market, early on in your career you will be on a level playing field with those who have graduated with a

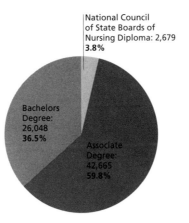

Nursing Graduates by Degree for Year 2000

BSN or from diploma schools. At that point, you can work almost anywhere an RN can work, matching your interests and abilities with the settings of your choice. Hospitals and other clinical arenas, long-term and sub-acute settings, community-based venues such as surgical centers, pioneer practices and well established clinics or physician's offices are all open to you. You can choose some specialty practice areas as well. Most hospitals, both urban and rural, have opportunities for registered nurses in all units including pediatrics, surgery, geriatrics, operating rooms and emergency rooms.

Certain areas of nursing, such as public health nursing, military career officers, management, administration, teaching and research require that you go back to school for a BSN degree. The beauty of an associate degree is that these specialties can open up to you simply by your adding two more years of schooling to your existing credits. With a BSN, you will then be able to study for an Advanced Practice nursing degree, or a master's degree, which opens many doors to more specialized professional options, including nurse practitioner, nurse midwife and specialist practices in family, acute care, pediatrics, neonatology, anesthesia and nursing informatics.

If you are seeking a career in nursing and you opt for an associate degree, you will have every opportunity to do what nurses for centuries before you have been doing — ministering to the ill and promoting health while making a measurable difference in the lives of patients. What's important is that today's prospective nurse has options — options that will undoubtedly lead to opportunity. Whatever your choice, I wish you all the best in preparing yourself for this wonderful career.

Marilyn A. Kaufmann is the Chair of the Nursing Program at Lakeshore Technical College in Cleveland, Wisconsin. She holds a bachelor's of science summa cum laude from the University of Wisconsin — Eau Claire, a master's degree in public health from the University of Minnesota and a PhD in Nursing from the University of Wisconsin in Milwaukee. Prior to coming to Lakeshore Technical College, Dr. Kaufmann was Director of Nursing in a long term care facility in Manitowoc, WI, administrator of a home health care agency, also in Manitowoc, and a staff nurse at various locations.

The following practice areas can be accessed with an associate's degree:

Cardiology	Long Term Care	Pediatric Palliative Care
Critical Care	Military	Perioperative
Emergency Room	Neonatal	(Operating Room)
Flight Trauma	Obstetrics	Psychiatric
Forensic	Occupational Health	Rehabilitation
Geriatric	Oncology	Urology
Home Care	Palliative Care/Hospice	
Industry	Pediatric	

challenges through time

In the twentieth century, nursing, as the largest healthcare profession in America, evolved from home visiting and community-based care to hospital- and institution-based care, and then back again to an increased emphasis on community care as patients experience shorter and shorter stays in the hospital. In addition, the creation of the nurse practitioner role gave birth to an advanced practice nurse, who joined the ranks of nurse-midwives and nurse anesthetists as professionals with expanded responsibilities and scope of care.

By Deborah S. Walker, DNSc, CNM, CS, FNP, Executive Secretary, American College of Nurse-Midwives, Assistant Professor and Coordinator, Nurse-Midwifery Education Program, University of Michigan School of Nursing

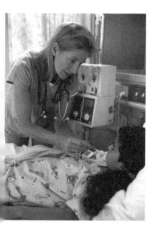

Since the beginning of modern nursing, nurses have made important contributions to health-care delivery by caring for the wounded and emotionally scarred on the front lines, often without adequate supplies and at great personal danger. During the Depression, they organized soup kitchens and led educational efforts to help families create inexpensive but nutritious meals. Nurses have also made important contributions to the health of women and children. In fact, the first organized prenatal care in this country was delivered by nurses. Mary Breckingridge, a nurse-midwife, demonstrated the positive impact nurse-midwives could make on maternal and neonatal mortality among impoverished families in the hills of Kentucky. And let us not forget the important contributions Margaret Sanger, a nurse, made to women's healthcare by opening the nation's first birth control clinic in Brooklyn, New York.

Caring is one of the most valuable attributes nursing has to offer. It is through caring that nurses enhance human dignity and ease suffering. Throughout the twentieth century, nurses embraced the latest healthcare changes and have met the challenges admirably. They learned how to care in new ways by becoming proficient in operating increasingly sophisticated technology, taking on ever — increasing responsibility for care and administering an ever-growing number of new treatments to save lives and heal wounded bodies, while also attending to the human spirit as well.

In addition to advances in the direct care provided by nurses, nursing as a profession matured in the twentieth century. Doctorally prepared nurses increased in numbers as did the number of doctoral programs in nursing. Increasingly throughout the century, nurses contributed to the expanding body of nursing and healthcare knowledge through investigations conducted by nurse researchers.

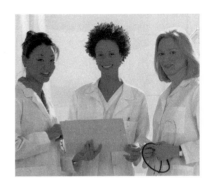

As the new millennium unfolds, other large challenges and opportunities face the profession. In addition to continuing to uphold high standards of patient care, one such challenge confronting the profession is the need to increase the visibility, respect, and recognition of nursing while maintaining its important role in healthcare delivery and research. Nursing, in many respects, is an invisible profession to the public. It has become increasingly difficult in healthcare settings to distinguish amongst healthcare providers, leading to increased confusion among those served. When nursing is visible, it is too often portrayed inaccurately. Nurses, themselves, often feel reluctant to communicate their worth to the public for social and political reasons, and may discount the important contributions they make. The result is relative invisibility for the profession and inaccurate perceptions that nurses are no more than 'physician extenders', 'handmaidens' or even the unrealistic characters portrayed on television. Nurse practitioners and nurse-midwives, in particular, are mistakenly perceived by the uninformed as physician "substitutes" or "midlevel providers" who are of lesser skills and quality and expendable when there are an adequate number of physicians on hand. In addition, little recognition is given to the similar but different conceptual frameworks from which the two separate professions derive. Medicine is concerned with diagnosing and treating illnesses; nursing is concerned with both of these, as well as the patient's response to both health and illness, including the environment and family. Nurses cannot substitute for physicians nor physicians for nurses. They provide complementary care.

Another challenge faced is the small role nurses have in crucial public discourse about healthcare and major social issues. It is here where nursing could have a significant impact on the public's health. The numbers alone suggest nurses could have enormous political clout and influence on the healthcare system of this country. But nursing's collective voice is often too soft, because too many in the profession don't get involved. But silence can be dangerous, because in this cost-cutting healthcare environment, silent nurses run the risk of being devalued and susceptible to budget cuts. Even with the current nursing shortage, if nurses do not have a strong voice and continue to champion the high quality care they provide, they could be replaced by unlicensed technicians as one solution to the shortage. All nurses, from staff nurses to academic researchers, must be seen and heard in public discussions on healthcare in order to maintain the excellent quality of care for which they have been singled out, and to maintain the reputation the profession has earned.

In the future, nurses will continue to face many challenges and must commit themselves on several fronts. All is not dark and bleak, as our nursing foremothers have laid an excellent foundation from which to continue to build the profession. A long-time hurdle facing the predominantly female profession is nursing's lack of power compared to that of physicians and hospital administrators. But as women continue to make inroads across the board, this more traditional issue will increasingly fade away. In addition, public opinion polls (if they continue to garner results in nursing's favor) are an additional factor helping to make this perception fade away. For example, a 1999 Gallup poll found that nurses are among the most trusted professionals by the public. Nurses will remain in a favorable position with the public if they continue to chip away at the fragmentation of care that exists in the healthcare profession. Nurses are in an ideal position to accomplish this, given their holistic view of healthcare. Ideally, those entering the profession will see nursing in a realistic light and embrace its continued efforts on all fronts. If so, both new and seasoned nurses can continue to provide high quality care while earning the respect of the public, policymakers and patients they serve, as well as influencing the direction and quality of healthcare in this new millennium.

Dr. Deborah S. Walker is the Executive Secretary of the American College of Nurse-Midwives in Washington, DC. Currently, she is Assistant Professor and Coordinator of the Nurse-Midwifery Education Program at the University of Michigan in Ann Arbor. She practices as a Certified Nurse-Midwife at North Campus Family Health Services in Ann Arbor, MI. Dr. Walker received a Master of Science in Nursing and Midwifery from the University of Minnesota in 1989 and a Doctor of Nursing Science from the University of California, Los Angeles in 1994. She has received numerous honors and recognition including the Excellence in Writing-Best Paper Award from the Journal of Nurse-Midwifery *and the University of Michigan Agenda for Women-Career Development Award.*

organizations
and resources

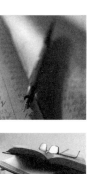

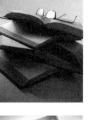

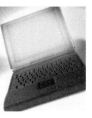

organizations and resources

A

Academy of Medical-Surgical Nurses (AMSN)
E. Holly Avenue, Box 56
Pitman, NJ 08071-0056
(856) 256-2323

Advanced Practice Nurse Journal (APNSCAN)
33 Main Street
Old Saybrook, CT 06475
860-395-0512

American Academy of Ambulatory Care Nursing (AAACN)
E. Holly Avenue, Box 56
Pitman, NJ 08071-0056
(856) 256-2350

American Academy of Nurse Practitioners (AANP)
P.O. Box 12846
Austin, TX 78711
(512) 442-4262

American Assembly for Men in Nursing (AAMN)
11 Cornell Road
Latham, NY 12110
(518) 782-9400 x346

American Association of Critical-Care Nurses (AACN)
101 Columbia
Aliso Viejo, CA 92656
(800) 899-2226

American Association for the History of Nursing (AAHN)
P.O. Box 175
Lanoka Harbor, NJ 08734
(609) 693-7250

American Association of Diabetes Educators (AADE)
100 West Monroe Street, Suite 400
Chicago, IL 60603
(800) 338-3633

American Association of Legal Nurse Consultants (AALNC)
4700 W. Lake Avenue
Glenview, IL 60025
(847) 375-4713

American Association of Managed Care Nurses (AAMCN)
P.O. Box 4975
Glen Allen, VA 23058-4975
(804) 747-9698

American Association of Office
Nurses (AAON)
109 Kinderkamack Road
Montvale, NJ 07645
(201) 391-2600

American Association of
Neuroscience Nurses (AANN)
4700 W. Lake Avenue
Glenview, IL 60025
(888) 557-2266
(847) 375-4733

American Association of Nurse
Anesthetists (AANA)
222 S. Prospect Avenue
Park Ridge, IL 60068
(847) 692-7050

The American Association of Nurse
Attorneys (TAANA)
7794 Grow Drive
Pensacola, FL 32514
(850) 474-3646
(877) 538-2262

American Association of
Occupational Health Nurses
(AAOHN)
2920 Brandywine Road, Suite 100
Atlanta, GA 30341
(770) 455-7757

American Association of Spinal
Cord Injury Nurses (AASCIN)
75-20 Astoria Boulevard
Jackson Heights, NY 11370
(718) 803-3782

American College of Health Care
Administrators (ACHCA)
1800 Diagonal Road, Suite 355
Alexandria, VA 22314
(703) 739-7900
(888) 88-ACHCA

American College of Nurse-
Midwives (ACNM)
818 Connecticut Avenue NW
Suite 900 Washington, DC 20006
(202) 728-9860

American College of Nurse
Practitioners (ACNP)
503 Capitol Court NE, Suite 300
Washington, DC 20002
(202) 546-4825

American Nephrology
Nurses' Association (ANNA)
E. Holly Avenue, Box 56
Pitman, NJ 08071-0056
(856) 256-2320

American Nurses
Association (ANA)
600 Maryland Avenue SW,
Suite 100 West
Washington, DC 20024
(202) 651-7000
(800) 274-4262

American Nurses Credentialing
Center (ANCC)
600 Maryland Avenue SW,
Suite 100 West
Washington, DC 20024
(202) 651-7000
(800) 284-2378

American Organization of Nurse
Executives (AONE)
325 Seventh Street NW
Washington, DC 20004
(202) 626-2240

American Psychiatric Nurses'
Association (APNA)
2107 Wilson Boulevard, Suite 300A
Arlington, VA 22201-3042
(703) 243-2443

American Society of Ophthalmic
Registered Nurses (ASORN)
P.O. Box 193030
San Francisco, CA 94119
(415) 561-8513

American Society of Pain
Management Nurses (ASPMN)
7794 Grow Drive
Pensacola, FL 32514
(888) 34-ASPMN

American Society for Parenteral and
Enteral Nutrition (ASPEN)
8630 Fenton Street, Suite 412
Silver Spring, MD 20910
(301) 587-6315
(800) 727-4567

American Society of PeriAnesthesia
Nurses (ASPAN)
10 Melrose Avenue, Suite 110
Cherry Hill, NJ 08003-3696
(877) 737-9696

American Society of Plastic Surgical
Nurses (ASPSN)
E. Holly Avenue, Box 56
Pitman, NJ 08071-0056
(856) 256-2340

Association of Camp Nurses
8504 Thorsonveien NE
Bemidji, MN 56601
(218) 586-2633

Association of Community Health
Nursing Educators (ACHNE)
11 Cornell Road
Latham, NY 12110
(850) 474-8821, ext. 289

Association of Nurses in
AIDS Care (ANAC)
11250 Roger Bacon Drive, Suite 8
Reston, VA 20190-5202
(703) 925-0081
(800) 260-6780

Association for Pediatric Oncology
Nurses (APON)
4700 W. Lake Avenue
Glenview, IL 60025-1485
(847) 375-4724

Association of periOperative
Registered Nurses (AORN)
2170 S. Parker Road, Suite 300
Denver, CO 80231
(303) 755-6300
(800) 755-2676

Association for Professionals
in Infection Control and
Epidemiology, Inc. (APIC)
1275 K Street NW, Suite 1000
Washington, DC 20005-4006
(202) 789-1890

Association of Rehabilitation
Nurses (ARN)
4700 W. Lake Avenue
Glenview, IL 60025-1485
(847) 375-4710
(800) 229-7530

Association of Women's Health,
Obstetric, and Neonatal Nurses
(AWHONN)
2000 L Street NW, Suite 740
Washington, DC 20036
(800) 673-8499

D

Dermatology Nurses'
Association (DNA)
E. Holly Avenue, Box 56
Pitman, NJ 08071
(856) 256-2330

Developmental Disabilities Nurses
Association (DDNA)
P.O. Box 2749
Eugene, Oregon 97402
(800) 888-6733

E

Emergency Nurses Association
(ENA)
915 Lee Street
Des Plaines, IL 60016-6569
(800) 900-9659

H

Honor Society of Nursing, Sigma Theta Tau International
550 W. North Street
Indianapolis, IN 46202
(317) 634-8171
(888) 634-7575

Hospice & Palliative Nurses Association (HPNA)
Penn Center West One, Suite 229
Pittsburgh, PA 15276
(412) 787-9301

I

International Association of Forensic Nurses (IAFN)
E. Holly Avenue, Box 56
Pitman, NJ 08071-0056
(856) 256-2425

International Nurses Society on Addictions (IntNSA)
1500 Sunday Drive, Suite 102
Raleigh, NC 27607
(919) 783-5871

International Society of Nurses in Genetics, Inc. (ISONG)
7 Haskins Road
Hanover, NH 03755
(603) 643-5706

International Society of Psychiatric-Mental Health Nurses (ISPN)
1211 Locust St.
Philadelphia, PA 19107
(800) 826-2950

International Council of Nurses
3, Place Jean Marteau
1201 — Geneva Switzerland
41-22-908-01-00

Intravenous Nurses Society (INS)
Fresh Pond Square
10 Fawcett St.
Cambridge, MA 02138
(617) 441-3008

M

Midwest Nursing Research Society (MNRS)
4700 W. Lake Avenue
Glenview, IL 60025
(847) 375-4711

N

National Association for Home Care (NAHC)
228 Seventh Street SE
Washington, DC 20003
(202) 547-7424

National Association of Neonatal Nurses (NANN)
4700 W. Lake Avenue
Glenview, IL 60025-1485
(800) 451-3795

National Association of Nurse Practitioners in Women's Health (NPWH)
503 Capitol Court NE, Suite 300
Washington, DC 20002
(202) 543-9693

National Association of Orthopaedic Nurses (NAON)
E. Holly Avenue, Box 56
Pitman, NJ 08071-0056
(856) 256-2310

National Association of Pediatric Nurse Associates and Practitioners (NAPNAP)
1101 Kings Highway North, Suite 206
Cherry Hill, NJ 08034
(856) 667-1773

National Association of School Nurses (NASN)
P.O. Box 1300
Scarborough, ME 04070-1300
(207) 883-2117

National Black Nurses Association (NBNA)
8630 Fenton Street, Suite 330
Silver Spring, MD 20910
(301) 589-3200

National Federation of Licensed Practical Nurses, Inc. (NFLPN)
893 US Highway 70 West, Suite 202
Garner, NC 27529
(919) 779-0046
(800) 948-2511

National Gerontological Nursing Association (NGNA)
7794 Grow Drive
Pensacola, FL 32514
(850) 473-1174
(800) 723-0560

National Institute of Nursing Research (NINR)
Building 31B
Rm 5B10, MSC 2178
31 Center Drive
Bethesda, MD 20892-2178
(301) 496-0207

National League for Nursing (NLN)
61 Broadway, 33rd Floor
New York, NY 10006
(212) 363-5555
(800) 669-1656

National Nursing Staff Development Organization (NNSDO)
7794 Grow Drive
Pensacola, FL 32514
(800) 489-1995

National Student Nurses Association (NSNA)
555 West 57th Street, Suite 1327
New York, NY 10019
(212) 581-2211

National Organization for Associate Degree Nursing (N-OADN)
11250 Roger Bacon Drive, Suite 8
Reston, VA 20190
(703) 437-4377

NursingHands.com
60 East 56th Street, 5th Floor
New York, NY 10022
(212) 888-4262

O

Oncology Nursing Society (ONS)
501 Holiday Drive
Pittsburgh, PA 15220-2749
(412) 921-7373

P

Preventive Cardiovascular Nurses Association (PCNA)
613 Williamson Street, Suite 205
Madison, WI 53703
(608) 250-2440

R

Respiratory Nursing Society (RNS)
11 Cornell Road
Latham, NY 12110
(518) 782-9400, ext 286

S

Society of Gastroenterology Nurses and Associates (SGNA)
401 N. Michigan Avenue
Chicago, IL 60611-4267
(312) 321-5165
(800) 245-7462

Society of Otorhinolaryngology and Head-Neck Nurses (SOHN)
116 Canal Street, Suite A
New Smyrna Beach, FL 32168
(904) 428-1695

Society of Pediatric Nurses (SPN)
7794 Grow Drive
Pensacola, FL 32514
(800) 723-2902

Society of Trauma Nurses (STN)
PMB 193
2743 S. Veterans Parkway
Springfield, IL 62704
(217) 787-3281

Society of Urological Nurses and
Associates (SUNA)
E. Holly Avenue, Box 56
Pitman, NJ 08071-0056
(856) 256-2335
(888) TAP-SUNA

Society for Vascular Nursing (SVN)
7794 Grow Drive
Pensacola, FL 32514
(850) 474-6963
(888) 536-4786

V

Visiting Nurse Associations of
America (VNAA)
11 Beacon Street, Suite 910
Boston, MA 02108
(617) 523-4042

W

Wound, Ostomy and Continence
Nurses Society (WOCNS)
4700 W. Lake Avenue
Glenview, IL 60025
(866) 615-8560
(888) 224-WOCN